TABLE OF CONTENTS

Top 20 Test Taking Tips

1. Carefully follow all the test registration procedures
2. Know the test directions, duration, topics, question types, how many questions
3. Setup a flexible study schedule at least 3-4 weeks before test day
4. Study during the time of day you are most alert, relaxed, and stress free
5. Maximize your learning style; visual learner use visual study aids, auditory learner use auditory study aids
6. Focus on your weakest knowledge base
7. Find a study partner to review with and help clarify questions
8. Practice, practice, practice
9. Get a good night's sleep; don't try to cram the night before the test
10. Eat a well balanced meal
11. Know the exact physical location of the testing site; drive the route to the site prior to test day
12. Bring a set of ear plugs; the testing center could be noisy
13. Wear comfortable, loose fitting, layered clothing to the testing center; prepare for it to be either cold or hot during the test
14. Bring at least 2 current forms of ID to the testing center
15. Arrive to the test early; be prepared to wait and be patient
16. Eliminate the obviously wrong answer choices, then guess the first remaining choice
17. Pace yourself; don't rush, but keep working and move on if you get stuck
18. Maintain a positive attitude even if the test is going poorly
19. Keep your first answer unless you are positive it is wrong
20. Check your work, don't make a careless mistake

Anatomy

Mammary gland development

Fetal

The mammary gland of the fetus goes through developmental stages related to the age of the embryo and its length from crown to rump. At about week 4, when the fetus is approximately 4 mm long, a mammary streak is observed. This streak becomes a milk line or ridge by week 5. The parenchyma cells of the mammary gland begin to proliferate at week 6. Embryonic development of the mammary gland is characterized by in growth of the outer layer of the embryo, the ectoderm, into the middle or mesoderm layer. This results in the following stages: a globular stage at weeks 7 to 8 (fetal length approximately 11-25 mm), a cone stage at week 9 (25 to 30 mm long), sprouting of epithelial buds between weeks 10 and 12 (up to 68 mm in length), lobular indentation buds and notching about week 13 (up to 8 cm long), and branching of these buds into epithelial strips about week 15 or 16 (length approximately 10 cm). These buds correspond to later secretory alveoli. Canals develop during weeks 20 to 32; this development is aided by placental hormones crossing into the fetal circulation around week 28. Weeks 32-40 are the end-vesicle stage of fetal mammary gland development.

The end-vesicle, or nipple, development stage of the fetus is the last phase of fetal mammary gland development prior to birth. This stage occurs during weeks 32 to 40 of embryonic development. At this point, the fetus is typically 35 to 50 cm in length. During previous developmental stages, the epidermis or outer layer of fetal skin initially thickens to form a primary bud. This bud then grows inward into the mesenchyma, which is the area that develops into connective tissues, blood, bone and the like. The indentation bud creates secondary buds branching from it, eventually forming a mammary pit or depression associated with lactiferous ducts. Initially the mammary pit is inverted but normally it elevates after further proliferation. By weeks 32 to 40, the alveoli are more lobular in appearance, mammary ducts and sebaceous glands come together around the epidermis, and colostrum or mammary fluid is present.

Prepubertal and pubertal

The mammary gland or breast develops in utero, before puberty, primarily up to age 2, and at puberty. It also undergoes later changes related to pregnancy and lactogenesis. After birth, both male and female newborns may secrete minute amounts of milk for up to a month due to stimulation of their mammary glands by placental hormones. During prepuberty, the female's mammary gland grows in relationship to the girl's physical growth. Before the onset of menses, mammary ducts extend into and branch in the mammary fat pad under the influence of systemic estrogen and growth hormone (GH) as well as local cellular interactions controlled by other hormones, such as insulin-like growth factor (IGF-1), human growth factor (HGF), and transforming growth factor-B (TGF-B). This process is known as organogenesis, and it is hastened just prior to puberty. Once menses occur, growth is primarily under system control of the hormones estrogen, progesterone, and possibly prolactin (PRL).

At puberty, phase I of breast development is characterized by a small elevation of the nipple but no visible glandular tissue or pigmentation of the areola. The second phase, which transpires at a mean age of 11.1 ($\pm$ 1.1) years, is indicated by projection of the nipple and breast and visible glandular tissue in the subareolar region. By a mean of 12.2 ($\pm$ 1.1) years, phase III usually occurs. This phase is characterized by enlargement of the breast, a wider and more pigmented areola and distinct glandular tissue. Phase IV typically commences by age 13; here the areola enlargement and increased pigmentation continue; in addition, the nipple and areola project distinctly from the rest of the breast. The last adolescent developmental stage (V) of the mammary glands occurs at a mean age of 15.3 years, during which the curvature of the breast is smoothed out.

Breast and mammary tissue location

The adult female normally has two breasts situated superficially between the second rib and the sixth intercostal cartilage, near the pectoralis major muscle, and horizontally just below the axillary line. The left breast is often larger. Each breast consists of skin, subcutaneous tissue, and a mass called the corpus mammae. Since the mammary gland originates in the fetus from the glandular milk line (sometimes called the galactic band), there are ridges of tissue in the adult female along the original milk lines. These lines extend from the groin area up through the breasts and axillae (armpits) into the upper inner arms. There are supernumerary nipples along these milk lines. Up to 6% of women develop hypermastia or visible mammary glands and nipples in other bodily regions along their remnant milk lines. Normal mammary glandular tissue also reaches into the axillary area, known as the tail of Spence, and is connected to the normal ductal system.

Breast abnormalities

There are several possible breast abnormalities. Hereditary absence of the breast, called amastia, is unusual. Presence of a nipple without breast tissue can occur and is called amazia. Presence of an extra nipple in addition to the normal breast is termed hyperthelia or polythelia, which has been associated with renal and other abnormalities. Some people have webbing in the midline region between their breasts, termed symmastia. When the breast is underdeveloped, the person is said to have breast hypoplasia, which is usually associated with underdevelopment of the pectoral muscles. One variant of hypoplasia is Poland Syndrome in which there is no pectoral muscle and there are chest and breast irregularities. Overdevelopment of one or both breasts is known as hyperplasia. Another possible abnormality is mammary tissue without a nipple, termed hyperadenia. The most common causes of acquired breast abnormalities include chest wall trauma from chest tube insertion in premature babies, skin burns to the chest wall area (including from radiation treatment), and childhood biopsies.

Corpus, papilla and areola mammae

The corpus mammae is the underlying mass of the breast. It includes the parenchyma, which is the totality of ductal, lobular and alveolar structures, and the stroma, which is comprised of the associated connective and fat tissues, blood vessels, nerves, and lymph system. There are alveolar glands, ductular branching alveoli, ducts, lactiferous sinuses, and lobular structures leading to the central nipple. Fat or adipose tissue provides support for the corpus mammae and its ductal system. The vast majority of women have lactiferous ducts and mammary tissues that extend into the armpit region; some also have these tissues near the midline or in the epigastria region. Both the nipple (the papilla mammae) and the circular pigmented area surrounding it (the areola mammae) are on the skin. The nipple is comprised of the extension of 10 to 20 milk ducts, smooth muscle fibers, sensory nerve endings, Meissner corpuscles, and sweat glands. The areola contains ductal openings for sebaceous, lactiferous, and sweat glands. The sebaceous glands of the areola are known as Montgomery glands.

Nipple erection and milk discharge

There are rings of smooth muscles in both the nipple and areola regions which aid in nipple erection and milk discharge. The dermal layers of both areas also incorporate many free nerve endings with multiple branches, and there are many areas of closely associated veins and arteries. The nipple becomes erect through changes in blood flow and contraction of the smooth muscles. The musculature of the breast is very fibrous and elastic allowing nipple erection and later emptying of the swollen ducts when a women nurses. Nipples can be stimulated to erection by touch, temperature changes, or sexual contact. The breast is supported by the ligaments of Cooper to retain its shape and not by supporting muscles.

Blood supply and lymphatic drainage

The breast receives blood primarily from the internal mammary and the lateral thoracic arteries. The intermammary artery supplies about 60% of the blood. Intercostal, axillary and subclavian arteries also provide a small blood supply to the area. The more reddish color of the nipple is due in large part to this blood supply. Veins carry blood from the same regions and there is a circulus venosus or anastomotic ring of veins around the nipple base. There are lymph capillaries in the breast connective tissue that drain primarily into the axillary nodes. There is also a small amount of drainage into the parasternal nodes in the thoracic cavity, the intermammary nodes connecting to the other breast, and nodes in the liver, the intraabdominal region, and the subclavicular area.

Innervation

The nipple and areola regions of the breast are innervated by both autonomic and sensory nerves branching from the fourth through sixth intercostal nerves. The supraclavicular nerves also innervate the area. The nipple contains norepinephrine-rich nerve fibers; norepinephrine is the principle sympathetic neurotransmitter. The corpus mammae are innervated by autonomic fibers to a lesser extent. Cutaneous nerves radiate toward the nipple. When sensory nerve fibers are stimulated, the hormones adenohypophyseal prolactin and neurohypophyseal oxytocin send messages to the hypothalamus in the brain, which controls involuntary reflexes. Norepinephrine is also liberated locally to cause muscular relaxation through stimulation of adrenergic receptors.

Morphological mammary gland changes

During menstrual cycle

Phases of the menstrual cycle correspond with morphological changes in the mammary gland. During phase I, days 3 to 7 of the menstrual cycle, the stroma is dense and cellular, the lumen is tight and, pale eosinophilic cells are the major epithelial cell observed. This is usually the only phase in which cells undergo mitosis or cell division. During phase II (8 to 14 days), the connective tissue stroma is more collagenous and the lumen is still defined; 3 types of epithelial cells radiating around the lumen are observed: luminar columnar basophilic cells, intermediate pale cells, and myoepithelial cells. Myoepithelial cells are epithelial contractile cells located at the base of secretory cells in mammary and other glands, also described as basal clear cells. In phase II, the myoepithelial cells have a hyperchromatic nucleus, whereas in later phases they show increasing vacuolization. The stroma looks loose and broken by phase III (days 15-20) and swollen with fluid by phase IV (days 21-27). In contrast, during these phases the lumen is open with increasing amounts of secretion, and phase IV is the period of active apocrine secretion from the luminal cell. Phase V, days 28 to 2, is characterized by dense cellular stoma, a swollen lumen, luminal basophilic and vacuolized basal cells and, occasionally, secretion.

During pregnancy

Pregnancy primarily impacts morphological changes in the mammary gland due to release of various hormones into circulation. The ductular, lobular and alveolar areas all grow. In the first month of pregnancy, release of estrogens causes ductular sprouting and some lobular development, which, during the second month, is evidenced by increased pigmentation of the nipple and areola, dilation of surface veins, and weightiness in the area. The first trimester is characterized by rapid proliferation of these ductal and lobular structures; shrinking of the relative adipose tissue; and permeation of lymphocytes, plasma cells, and eosinophils into the area. Epithelial cell growth is augmented during the pregnancy through release of prolactin while other tissue types diminish. There is a transition toward lactogenesis and milk secretion.

During lactation and post-lactation

The distinguishing feature of the lactating mammary gland is the sizeable number of alveoli composed of cuboidal and myoepithelial cells present. These alveoli develop during the third trimester. Lactogenesis or milk secretion is regulated by prolactin, oxytocin, and the nervous system. The protein and fat portions of milk are created and released through slightly different mechanisms; protein is expelled directly whereas fatty

components must be released from the cytoplasm. The mammary gland regresses and milk manufacture stops if there is no sucking or removal of milk. This occurs because there is no stimulation of the neurohormonal mechanisms for prolactin release, blood vessels are constricted diminishing flow as well as access to oxytocin, and alveoli break down while fat and other connective tissues increase. There may be residual cords of epithelial cells but for the most part the mammary gland returns to the pre-pregnancy condition. This process is also known as involution.

Physical assessment for breastfeeding

The breast should be inspected for variations that could potentially affect ability to breastfeed. Conspicuous asymmetry between breasts can indicate inadequate glandular tissue in some women. Lactation can be affected by hypoplasia, lack of breast tissue, and broad spacing between breasts. Overdeveloped women may have to approach breastfeeding differently from others (such as lifting and holding the breast) which can affect the decision to nurse. The breast skin should be checked for variations in turgor and elasticity. The woman should be inspected for thickened areas suggestive of tumors, incisions that might indicate previous breast surgery, and possible nerve damage and structural abnormalities of the breast (like inversion). They should be queried about the occurrence of normal hormonal-responsive increases in breast size, swelling and tenderness.

Pinch test

The pinch test is normally part of the physical assessment of the breast for the woman wishing to breastfeed. It is a form of palpation in which the clinician compresses or palpates the areola between their forefinger and thumb behind the nipple base mimicking infant compression while breastfeeding. The pinch test assesses nipple function and should be done at regular intervals during pregnancy because functionality can change. Nipple function is classified as protraction, retraction, or inversion. Protraction, movement of the nipple forward during the test, is the normal functional reaction. Retraction means the nipple moves inward. A healthy infant with a robust suck can overcome minimal retraction and pull the nipple out, but if the nipple retracts into the areola, stretching of the nipple outward will be necessary to accomplish breastfeeding. Inversion is the situation in which a nipple is pulled into the areola on visual inspection alone. There are two versions of inversion: simple, in which manual pressure or cold can protract the nipple, and complete, which is unresponsive to pressure due to adhesions in the underlying connective tissue.

Oral cavity development in newborns

The facial and pharyngeal regions in the fetus initially develop from neural-crest cells and are further differentiated through endodermal cells that form the digestive tract. When the child is born, their mouth dimensions differ proportionately from an adult. The infant's mouth is short vertically, the lower jaw is smaller and further back, the hard palate is shorter and less arched than an adult's, fat pads are on both cheeks, and the tongue is in contact with the gums and roof of the mouth because of the small cavity. The infant has folds on the hard palate and swellings on the lip called eminences of the pars villosa, both of which aid the suckling reflex. The child's epiglottis is right under the soft palate (the two are much further apart in adults), which enables the infant to pass food directly into the esophagus. The larynx is also relatively high and easy to protect during swallowing.

Physiology and Endocrinology

Mammary gland development

The fetal stage of mammary gland development is known developmentally as embryogenesis. Mammogenesis is the development of the mammary gland to a functional state, including an increase in size and weight of the breast and the development of ducts and the glandular system. There are several periods when mammogenesis is prevalent, particularly during puberty and pregnancy, and the primary hormones involved are estrogen, progesterone, and prolactin. Lactogenesis, the initiation of milk synthesis, is generally regarded as divided into two stages. The second stage occurs 3 to 8 days after birth. During this stage, abundant amounts of milk are secreted as a result of a drop in maternal progesterone. Galactopoiesis is lactation or the maintenance of milk production directly thereafter under autocrine control and prolactin (PRL) and oxytocin regulation. About 40 days after breastfeeding stops, involution or decreased milk secretion occurs coinciding with PRL withdrawal.

Essential physiological and endocrine factors
An adipose or fat tissue pad must be present to sustain ductal proliferation; this pad normally develops during midgestation. The female secondary hormone estrogen must also be available; its augmentation during puberty contributes to mammary development at that time. Cells having estrogen receptors enhance ductal cell propagation through release of a paracrine factor. An intact pituitary gland capable of secreting growth hormone (GH), which also promotes release of insulin-like growth factor 1 (IGF-1), is required. The arrangement of mammary ducts and buds is controlled by transforming growth factor beta (TGF-*B*). Progesterone (PGR) initiates ductal side branching, and prolactin (PRL) is necessary for complete alveolar expansion. Other hormones, such as the growth factor heregulin (HER), appear to play roles as well.

Mammogenesis

Before and during puberty and the menstrual cycle
Boys and girls both show ductal enlargement proportionate to their growth until just prior to puberty. At that point, the duct system proliferates rapidly in the female under the influence of estrogen. Other hormones such as adrenocorticotropic hormone (ACTH) and thyroid-stimulating hormone (TSH) appear to affect breast growth somewhat during prepuberty as well, and transmembrane glycoproteins called integrins play a role in regulation of cell growth and differentiation. At puberty, ducts, terminal intralobular ductules, and alveoli proliferate extensively from epithelial and underlying myoepithelial cells and the connective tissue of the stroma becomes organized. Estrogens induced during the menstrual cycle contribute to formation of epithelial sprouts as well as lobular swelling and secretory matter (also influenced by progesterone). In the luteal stage, there is also increased blood flow in the breast. Once the menstruation part of the cycle begins, these changes subside somewhat but tend to contribute to continued mammary growth until about age 30.

During pregnancy
During pregnancy, placental and luteal hormones augment ductal sprouting, branching, and formation of lobules. Human placental lactogen (HPL), prolactin, and human corticotropin (hCG) promote growth while estrogens affect

sprouting and progesterone promotes lobular formation and prevents milk secretion prior to term. These hormones prime the breast for lactation in several ways. They can send messages to the hypothalamus to inhibit other hormones and factors, influencing adenohypophysis, or directly stimulate development of the ducts, lobules, and alveoli of the mammary gland. An important factor under hypothalamic control is prolactin-inhibiting factor, which is depressed to allow prolactin synthesis and liberation enhancing direct breast stimulation. Prolactin is necessary for comprehensive gland development. Other metabolic hormones are increased such as cortical, insulin, thyroid, parathyroid, and growth hormones. Material resembling colostrum is present from approximately the third month of gestation. Transforming growth factor beta (TGF-B) regulates pattern formation.

Postpartum preparation for lactation

Stage I lactogenesis begins during the last trimester of pregnancy and continues until about day 3 postpartum. The constituents of milk are manufactured during the pregnancy and released under stimulation by prolactin after parturition. During the first few days after delivery, progesterone levels plummet while prolactin remains relatively constant. After that period, milk must be removed via infant suckling which induces oxytocin production and release to maintain secretion. About day 2 or 3 postpartum, stage II begins and is characterized by increasing blood flow, oxygen and glucose absorption, citrate levels, and plasma a-lactalbumin. Abundant milk production begins. Glucose, free phosphate and calcium concentrations also increase, and the pH falls.

Human prolactin

Levels and functions
Human prolactin, a pituitary hormone, is present in both males and females. In males and prepubertal or postmenopausal females, prolactin levels are in the range of 2 to 8 ng/mL. In menstruating females, the average concentration of prolactin is 10 ng/mL; this increases dramatically during pregnancy (~200 ng/mL) and is even more striking in amniotic fluid (possibly 10^4 ng/mL). When new birth mothers breastfeed, the initial rise to about 400 ng/mL decreases during the first year but remains higher than those who do not breastfeed. The newborn child does absorb some of the prolactin. Prolactin activates sodium/potassium adenosine triphosphatase which controls expression of milk protein genes. It affects the mammary glands' immune system, primarily by drawing in immunoglobulin A immunoblasts. The hormone also binds to membrane receptors on mammary epithelial cells to aid in the synthesis of messenger RNA associated with milk proteins. Plasma prolactin levels have been shown to affect coping mechanisms.

Control mechanisms during lactogenesis
Prolactin is a pituitary hormone, but its levels are controlled by other mechanisms as well. Prolactin levels can be inhibited by prolactin-inhibiting factor (PIF), which is in turn controlled by catecholamine levels under direction of the hypothalamus. Prolactin production is strongly stimulated by thyrotrophic-releasing hormone (TRH). A number of other pharmacologic agents either stimulate or suppress release of prolactin. Some of the more notable agents are the stimulant estrogen and the suppressor dopamine. The most powerful inducement of prolactin release is nipple or breast manipulation through infant suckling (or mechanical pumping devices). Other physiologic stimuli can

- 12 -

also affect release such as stress, sexual intercourse, or pregnancy. Prolactin concentrations are higher nocturnally than during the day. No direct correlation between the volume of milk and prolactin levels has been demonstrated.

Other hormones found during lactogenesis

Human placental lactogen (hPL) is a hormone whose levels rise during gestation just like prolactin and then plummet upon placental delivery. It originates from the chorionic membrane and is very similar structurally and immunologically to the other important lactogenic hormone, human growth hormone (hGH). hGH is released from anterior pituitary eosinophilic cells during lactation; it generally increases during suckling but is not essential for milk secretion. Oxytocin, which is present in both sexes, helps trigger lactation in women. Oxytocin is manufactured by hypothalamic cells, and its release is augmented by a number of neurological substances, such as serotonin and dopamine, and inhibited by others, like opiates and endorphins. Oxytocin enhances lactation by producing a soothing effect and lowering blood pressure and pulse rates, thus making it easier to interface with the child.

Let-down reflex and neuroendocrine control of milk-ejection

The let-down reflex (also known as the ejection reflex) is the release of milk from alveoli and tinier milk ducts into the larger lactiferous ducts and sinuses upon suckling. It is due to oxytocin release from the pituitary gland. Oxytocin can also stimulate contractions in the uterus for delivery, and it can be discharged upon other sensory stimulation besides suckling, such as sight, touch, smell, or hearing. Oxytocin levels return to baseline (3.3 to 4.7 ng/mL) between milk-ejections, whereas prolactin levels are maintained. Maintenance of milk-ejection requires carrying neural responses to the brain and efferent release of endocrine substances. Tactile stimulation of the nipple area is the most important factor in lactation; receptors for both oxytocin and prolactin are located in the nipple. The intramammary pressure increases significantly in the initial days after delivery due, in large part, to release of relatively small amounts of oxytocin. Secretion of oxytocin, which also stimulates anterior pituitary hormones associated with milk secretion, continues for about a year. Prolactin levels go down but are still above baseline.

FIL and other adaptive responses

There is a whey protein in milk called the feedback inhibitor of lactation (FIL). FIL regulates secretion of milk components through autocrine inhibition in the lactating mammary gland. Its effects are directly related to its concentration, and FIL does not change milk composition. The mother adapts in a number of ways to lactation. Adipose tissue metabolism changes to provide milk that is rich in fats. The mother's intestine, liver and heart enlarge and become more complex during lactation to accommodate greater energy needs. Increased calcium needs are addressed through elevation in dihydroxycholecalciferol from late gestation through early lactation. Glucose production is also ramped up.

Computerized breast measurement

Computerized breast measurement (CBM) is a method of measuring milk synthesis without compromising the infant's breastfeeding pattern. CBM measures variations in breast volume during feeding as well as during pregnancy, volume of milk removed upon feeding, and the following parameters. The first parameter is the short-term rate of milk synthesis (S), defined as the increase in breast volume between feedings divided by the time between recordings. Another parameter is storage capacity (SC), described as the difference between maximum and minimum breast volumes during a 24-hour interval. Normal values for storage capacity are between 80 and 600 mL. Lastly, CBM can define the degree of fullness (F), which is the ratio between a specific breast volume and the storage capacity at that moment. CBM is more efficient than other methodologies like weighing the mother and infant, isotope dilution techniques, and expressing or removing milk by means other than suckling.

Mammary secretory cells

Phases during lactation

Mammary apocrine or secretory cells are in resting phases between periods of milk secretion. Cells become more differentiated structurally during pregnancy. They demonstrate synthesis and secretion of proteins and fat during early stages of lactation as illustrated by protein caps, surface lipid droplets, and polarization of the secretory cell. Proteins, lactose, lipids, and ions are enclosed in secretory vesicles and extruded at the cell surface into the alveoli to begin the process of milk synthesis. Typically a resting cell passes through secretory phases of beginning milk synthesis to spontaneous and provoked milk secretion periods and then returns to another resting phase.

Structures and functions

Secretory cells in the mammary gland consist of the nucleus, cytosol, endoplasmic reticulum, mitochondria, and Golgi apparatus. The nucleus contains the genetic material of the cell and is the place where deoxyribonucleic acid (DNA) and ribonucleic acid (RNA) are synthesized. Cytosol, also known as the particle-free supernatant, is the fluid part of the cytoplasm excluding organelles and other structures; it is the portion where a number of enzymes and cofactors associated with milk production are located. The mitochondria are small bodies in the cytoplasm that provide energy, through adenosine triphosphate (ATP), and facilitate respiratory activity in the cell; they enlarge and become more active during lactation. The Golgi apparatus and the endoplasmic reticulum (as well as the cell membranes) are considered part of the microsomal fraction of the cell whose primary purpose is to aid synthesis of the constituents of milk. Some functions of the Golgi apparatus are lactose synthesis and packaging while the endoplasmic reticulum synthesizes proteins, triglycerides, and phospholipids.

Milk production and secretion into mammary alveolus

There are 5 ways milk can be produced and secreted into the mammary alveolus. Four of these pathways occur transcellularly or within the cell. One of these is exocytosis or release to the cell surface of lactose and milk proteins through vesicles originating in the Golgi apparatus; this pathway involves calcium, phosphate, and citrate ions. Another conduit is the excretion of milk lipids at the surface as milk fat globules. A third is the leakage of water and sodium, potassium, and chloride ions across the outer membrane. The fourth transcellular pathway is the pinocytosis and exocytosis of immunoglobulins and possibly other plasma proteins; pinocytosis is the inward pinching of a cell membrane to form an internal vesicle and take in fluids. Milk synthesis and secretion is also aided via a paracellular pathway in which plasma components and leukocytes can pass from the capillary between cells into the mammary alveolus.

Milk synthesis and lactation

Carbohydrates and associated pathways
The two most important carbohydrates related to milk synthesis are glucose and lactose. Glucose is the major resource for energy, carbon molecules, and milk output. When glucose and uridine diphosphogalactose react, lactose (plus uridine diphosphate or UDP) results. The reaction's catalyst is the whey protein lactalbumin, which spikes after delivery due to a drop in progesterone and estrogen concentrations. Lactose is a carbohydrate found only in milk. During lactogenesis, the concentration of lactose increases 2 to 3 days postpartum from a baseline of approximately 80 mmol/L to about 160 mmol/L and the difference represents the lactose output. Glucose concentration and output also increases at the same time.

Fats and associated pathways
Fats are synthesized from carbohydrates. The alveolar cells can assemble long-chain fatty acids from carbohydrates in blood plasma, short-chain fatty acids primarily from acetate, and triglycerides from pentose (or obtain them directly from the plasma). Glycerol is taken into the cells from the capillaries and broken down by an enzyme called lipoprotein lipase. Glycerides are synthesized into triglycerides via the catalyst palmitoyl-coenzyme A (CoA) 1-glycerol-3-phosphate palmitoyl transferase. Both enzymes spike after delivery under the influence of prolactin and insulin. Fats are synthesized at the endoplasmic reticulum by esterification of fatty acids. Triglycerides form fat droplets eventually released at the cell surface as milk fat globules (MFG) enclosed in membranes. The MFG serve to maintain emulsion stability of the milk.

Proteins and associated pathways
The three important milk proteins, casein, a-lactalbumin, and B-lactalbumin, are secreted only during lactation. They are manufactured from free amino acids in secretory cells on the ribosomes of the endoplasmic reticulum under the stimulation of prolactin, insulin and cortisol. The proteins travel to the Golgi complex where they become glycosylated and phosphorylated and then are released via secretory vesicles through exocytosis. Release of proteins (as well as fats, lactose, citrate, calcium and phosphate) is unidirectional from the cell to the alveolar lumen, whereas other ions, water, and glucose can permeate the membrane in both directions. A-lactalbumin is required for lactose synthesis using galactosyl transferase. Casein is complexed with calcium and phosphate in electrically charged micelles. Protein can also be secreted via protein capping.

Water, ions and other substances in lactation

Human milk has the same osmotic pressure and concentration of substances in it as plasma, but the high levels of lactose in human milk are balanced by lower concentrations of ions. Milk is also positively charged relative to fluids within the cells, while the cell membrane is negatively charged. Fluids inside the cells and in the milk both maintain a 3:1 gradient of potassium to sodium ions. After delivery, the main ion found to increase in concentration and output in milk is citrate. The mechanism of citrate secretion is presently unclear, but it is the primary buffering system in milk (along with phosphate to a lesser extent). Calcium levels and release increase postpartum but are primarily associated with casein. Milk also contains some milk enzymes (most notably lipase which breaks down triglycerides), proteolytic enzymes, protease inhibitors, the iron-binding protein lactoferrin, and white blood cells. The white blood cells include macrophages, which probably aid in immune defense through release of secretory IgA immediately following delivery, and immune leukocytes.

Physiologic changes during involution

Typical milk volume during lactation is 600 mL/day. When a child is being weaned, some changes in milk composition occur as milk volumes fall below about 400 mL/day. In particular, lactose levels decrease while milk protein, chloride, and sodium levels increase. During measured weaning from breastfeeding, citrate, phosphate, calcium, and glucose concentrations diminish while fat, potassium, and magnesium levels are higher. Physiologically during involution or a return to normal size after lactation, the secretory epithelial cells experience apoptosis and programmed cell death initially. Then the extracellular milieu is adjusted, interfaces between mesenchymal and epithelial cells are modified, more cells undergo apoptosis, and the majority of mammary epithelium dies and is absorbed.

Lactation amenorrhea

Lactation amenorrhea, also known as postpartum ovarian refractoriness, is the absence of menstruation during lactation. This phenomenon is probably due to changes resulting from nervous impulses from nipple stimulation. These include an elevation in prolactin levels during the lactation period, alterations in ovarian hormone feedback mechanisms, hypothalamic suppression of gonadotropin-releasing hormone (Gn-RH), and the release of B-endorphin. Gn-RH influences release from the pituitary gland of both the follicle-stimulating hormone (FSH) and the luteinizing hormone (LH) involved in the menstrual cycle. Depressed levels of gonadotropin have been demonstrated in the initial weeks after delivery. Estradiol (E_2), an estrogenic hormone, remains at lower concentrations longer in women who are lactating as well.

Return of menstruation and ovulation

Non-nursing mothers usually experience a return to menstruation by the third month after delivery, with possible observation of menstruation 4 weeks postpartum. Forty percent of non-nursing mothers menstruate by 6 weeks after delivery, about two-thirds menstruate at 12 weeks, and 90% do so by 24 weeks postpartum. The return of ovulation percentages are less for the same time period, non-nursing mothers may have a shortened secretory phase, and their menses may be irregular. If they are amenorrheic, the return of ovulation tends to be delayed. On the other hand, in mothers who breastfeed exclusively, the return of menses is statistically low (up to 30%) 3 months postpartum and even at 6 months in at least half of the population. Initial menstruation is sometimes seen at 4 to 6 months postpartum. The frequency of breastfeeding affects the possibility of ovulation. For example, a woman who breast feeds 10 times a day has only a 1% chance of ovulating, which increases with fewer daily feeds. A longer interval before first menses increases the possibility of ovulation. The initial cycles may show insufficient luteal function.

Family planning during lactation

Pregnancy during breastfeeding
For women having unprotected intercourse after delivering a baby, the probability of pregnancy is significantly lowered with breastfeeding. A nonlactating woman with normal fertility has close to 100% chance of becoming pregnant within a year postpartum. Women who breastfeed show a lag period of at least 3 months after delivery in which pregnancy is improbable. Most nursing mothers can become pregnant by 2 years postpartum. If the breastfeeding

female has unprotected intercourse only during the period of lactation amenorrhea followed by later contraception, the probability of pregnancy within 2 years is less than 20%. Prolonged breastfeeding can also protract the period of lactational amenorrhea. Contraceptive use can suppress milk yield, while factors like night feedings and postponement of solids or other liquids can prolong the birth interval.

Breastfeeding can prolong the period of lactational amenorrhea. The lactational amenorrhea method (LAM), having unprotected sex only during the phase of lactation amenorrhea and then using some type of birth control, has been shown to be effective. Studies have shown protective rates greater than 98% at 6 months postpartum (pp) and over 80% at 2 years pp. About 19% of women using LAM have a cumulative risk of bleeding within 6 months after delivery, but the majority of these cycles are inovulatory. If the mother experiences bleeding during the first few months postpartum, other birth control measures are indicated. On the other hand, if she is amenorrheic at that time and fully breastfeeding the child, the chance of pregnancy is only about 2% until bleeding transpires.

<u>Natural measures for contraception</u>
Fertility can be predicted during lactation by basal temperature, cervical mucus, and cervical assessment. The basal body temperature is low during the relatively infertile period including menses, begins to rise around the period of ovulation and fertility, and then peaks before declining after the fertile period. Conception is impossible during the last phase. Cervical mucus, which conveys sperm to the egg for fertilization, is another predictor of menstrual phase and possible fertility. During ovulation and possible fertility, the mucus is wet and thick, but is dry and less penetrable by sperm in the phases prior to and after ovulation. Mucus is

detected on average about 2 months prior to first menses, but this parameter is often difficult to interpret. Another observation for natural family planning is to assess whether the cervix is open or closed; an open cervix indicates ovulation and possible fertility.

<u>Oral and other contraceptives</u>
Contraceptive use during lactation does not change milk composition, but it can suppress milk yield and subject the mother or infant to undesired effects. Therefore, the concentration of hormones in the preparation should be kept to no more than 2.5 mg 19-norprogestogen, 50 μg ethinyl estradiol, or 100 μg methanol. Generally the lactating mother is only started on contraceptives if she is bleeding, feeding infrequently (at least 6 hour intervals), using supplementation, and confirmed by physical examination as not being pregnant. Then she is either started immediately on the mini-pill or low-dose oral preparations, or she is given barrier-type contraceptives to use for 2 weeks, at which time pregnancy re-evaluation takes place before starting oral contraceptives. Injectable contraceptives such as medroxyprogesterone (Depo-Provera) or implants like the Norplant System (containing levonorgestre) are sometimes used without long-term side effects.

<u>Additional contraceptive methods</u>
The ovulation method (OM) for predicting ovulation can be quite effective during the first 6 months postpartum when full breastfeeding is used. There are a number of home ovulation tests that monitor daily estrone conjugates in urine samples. Intranasal use of a preparation of luteinizing hormone releasing hormone (LH-RH) appears promising for contraception. Barrier methods such as condoms, intrauterine devices (IUDs), cervical caps, diaphragms, and vaginal suppositories or creams are acceptable forms of contraception during this period

with varying degrees of effectiveness. Some studies advocate IUD insertion immediately upon or within several months of delivery, while others suggest an increased risk of perforation by the IUD in lactating women. Abstinence is an effective contraceptive method as well.

Milk composition during ovulatory menstrual cycles

Some constituents of mammary milk change in concentration during an ovulatory menstrual cycle in lactating women, while other components remain fairly constant. The main changes found are in the sodium and chloride concentrations, which both increase significantly the week after ovulation. In addition, potassium and lactose levels decrease in the same phase. These results suggest that ovulation increases the permeability of the mammary epithelium. These substantial changes are not observed in lactating women not undergoing ovulation, such as those in lactational amenorrhea, those whose cycles are not ovulatory, and those taking contraceptives.

Sexual arousal and activity during lactation

Physiological and psychological responses to lactation and coitus are very similar. During both, nipples are excited and become erect, the uterus contracts, the let-down or milk-ejection reflex can occur, the skin becomes warm and shows blood vessel dilation, and similar feelings are aroused. These responses are due to the fact that similar hormones are involved in lactation and intercourse. Sexual activity in lactating women is variable, but in general, it is resumed about a month after delivery. Some mothers are much more interested in sex while breastfeeding, while others are uninterested for the first few months. Most studies also indicate that more

mothers who breastfeed feel that their sexual relationship with the partner improves, not diminishes, upon resumption. The hormones associated with lactation can produce excessive vaginal dryness and possible painful intercourse primarily because progesterone produced during pregnancy hinders maturation of epithelial cells. Another issue can be triggering the milk-ejection reflex during sexual activity, which can be avoided by prior infant feeding or milk expression.

Nursing during pregnancy or tandem nursing

There is no reason to contraindicate nursing an infant if the mother becomes pregnant One major concern is the ability to provide enough nutrition for the newborn infant while the older child is still nursing, known as tandem nursing. In addition, a new mother, who never discontinued nursing the older child, will initially produce colostrum, which is important for the newborn but not the older child. When the mother becomes pregnant, spontaneous weaning often occurs, or the mother decides to wean because of breast and nipple pain. Some studies indicate that infants weaned during a new pregnancy have short-term reductions in growth rate compared to other weaning scenarios. Weaning should not be done hastily.

Breastfeeding does place additional demands on the mother for energy resources; she may require supplement intake, especially if pregnant. Breastfeeding also temporarily diminishes bone mineral density from calcium consumption and uses up fat stores. Vigorous infants who continue to feed during the mother's pregnancy still get nutritional and immunological benefits. Major concerns about breastfeeding while pregnant involve the fetus. There is an increased threat of fetal

- 18 -

loss or preterm labor in these mothers. Oxytocin liberated during breastfeeding can induce uterine contractions and loss of the fetus; additionally, nipple stimulation can trigger labor. High risk pregnancies, such as multiple fetuses, indicate weaning the infant.

Induced lactation, relactation, and inappropriate lactation

Induced lactation is the stimulation of lactation in a woman who has not been recently pregnant, such as an adoptive parent. Lactation can also be induced in a postmenopausal woman who has had a child through fertility techniques and hormone therapy. Relactation is the provocation of lactation in a woman who did give birth but did not nurse at that time or one who weaned an infant from breastfeeding and desires to start nursing again. Inappropriate lactation, also known as galactorrhea, is any situation in which unexpected lactation occurs. Inappropriate lactation includes lactation in women who have never had children, in men, in females who have terminated a pregnancy 3 or more months prior to the incident, and in women who weaned an infant at least 3 months in the past.

Induced lactation
Preparation of breasts: A woman preparing for induced lactation normally develops a schedule of nipple stimulation and milk expression (manually or with the assistance of a pumping device). The woman can also take hormones normally stimulated during pregnancy, principally estrogen, progesterone, and human placental lactogen. Typically she would take oral contraceptives that contain estrogen and progesterone, which are discontinued about a month before she wishes to lactate; the woman preparing for induced lactation would generally also use a pump for expression and take domperidone, an antidopaminergic drug, which can increase prolactin secretion

and induce lactation. Lactation usually begins after 1 to 6 weeks of preparation. Other choices to stimulate growth of the alveoli and ducts include conjugated estrogens.

Pharmacologic agents: There are a number of pharmacologic agents that can be used to induce prolactin secretion and lactation after stopping contraceptives or other methods of proliferation. Most agents are classified as galactogogues, agents that promote secretion of milk. Thyrotropin-releasing hormone (TRH) directly stimulates adenohypophyseal lactrotrophs, cells in the anterior pituitary that produce prolactin. Theophylline, which is present in tea and coffee, can also directly boost prolactin secretion. Several agents act by affecting PIF or prolactin-inhibiting factor. These include phenothiazines, like the sedative chlorpromazine, which suppresses PIF activity by decreasing hypothalamic levels of dopamine and catecholamine as well as metoclopramide, a dopamine antagonist. Other drugs that can increase prolactin secretion are growth hormone, which optimizes milk production; sulpiride, which potentiates hypothalamic prolactin-releasing hormone; and recombinant human growth hormones (hGHs), which act on prolactin receptors. Nasally-administered oxytocin can aid in the initial ejection response.

Prolactin secretion can be decreased by pharmacologic agents that either enhance the activity of or actually increase prolactin-inhibiting factor. L-Dopa suppresses prolactin secretion by augmenting the hypothalamic levels of the neurotransmitters dopamine and catecholamine, which in turn increase the activity of PIF. These types of agents may be important because prolactin secretion is affected by hypothalamic dopamine turnover. The ergot alkaloids ergocornine and ergocryptine directly inhibit the adenohypophyseal secretion of prolactin and may also act by increasing or prolonging the hypothalamus controlled activity of prolactin-inhibiting factor.

Composition of milk: The protein content of non-biologic milk obtained by induced lactation differs somewhat from normal biologic breast milk. Total protein has been shown to be significantly less during the first few days of nursing. Overall, the mean value for levels of *a*-lactalbumin has been shown to be slightly lower in induced-nursing mothers. The milk produced by induced lactation is closer in composition to real biologic milk than colostrum, however. Some studies have shown differences in ionic concentrations. If the breast is hyperstimulated, so-called low volume "galactorrhea milk" does appear to be extremely high in sodium content and low in potassium.

Physiological changes: A women nursing through induced lactation can experience irregular menstrual cycles, decreased menstrual flow, complete amenorrhea, or milk flow irregularities related to the menstrual cycle. Her breast may change in size and feel heavy or full. These women usually gain an average of 10-12 lbs. Depending on the method of nipple stimulation used prior to nursing; the breast may be sore and irritated. This soreness is more likely if hand-operated pumps are used than if electric pumps or manual stroking and massaging are utilized. If the adoptive mother is stressed or rigid after the baby's arrival, she may have difficulty lactating, mostly due to lack of the ejection reflex.

Nutritional supplementation for adoptive mothers
Once the baby arrives, the adoptive mother should restrict the infant's sucking to breastfeeding. The mother should breastfeed before she gives the child any other type of nutritional supplementation. Depending on the child's age and eating habits prior to adoption, supplementation is often indicated. Infants up to 1 year of age may need infant formula (or sometimes donor human milk but not whole milk) at a concentration of 20 kcal/oz. This preparation may be administered while breastfeeding using a dropper or supplementer or afterwards with a spoon, dropper, or cup. Rubber nipples or pacifiers confuse the infant and should not be used. Older children who are already eating solid foods can continue using a spoon.

Relactation
Reasons: Relactation is often used by mothers of sick or premature infants who could not be breastfed at birth. It may be indicated when an infant who was not formerly breastfed develops some type of allergy or food intolerance. Relactation is often utilized in order to return to breastfeeding with infants that were weaned prematurely because of health issues or illness involving either the mother or child. Another reason for relactation is the adoption of an infant (occurring during or after nursing a biological child). Relactation has been successful after a year post-lactation but is less likely in women who have undergone complete postpartum breast involution.

Drugs and devices: Some of the same drugs used for induced lactation are used to promote relactation. TRH, thyrotrophic-releasing hormone (known commercially as Thyroliberin), has been studied by several investigators to induce prolactin release and lactation and has been found useful. The procainamide derivatives metoclopramide and sulpiride have also been tried; results are inconclusive but there is some evidence that metoclopramide does increase milk volume. There are supplemental devices designed to provide extra nourishment to the infant while suckling; these include the Lact-Aid Trainer System and the

- 20 -

Supplemental Nursing System. These methods of supplementation or other complementary nourishment, such as formula or donor human milk, are often necessary in order to prevent infant starvation.

Cross-nursing

Cross-nursing is the occasional nursing of another woman's child while a mother is also nursing her own. This may occur as a result of some type of babysitting arrangement, as a means of stimulating lactation in adoptive nursing, when a woman's own baby is not providing enough stimulation, or when the mother of an immature baby makes use of someone else's infant to provoke milk production. These scenarios require private arrangements and are not well controlled. There are dangers to cross-nursing, in particular the risk of infection with human immunodeficiency virus (HIV) or other infectious agents, such as hepatitis or tuberculosis. There can also be psychological issues and differences in milk composition that may impact children of different ages. Historically cross-nursing was known as wet nursing.

Suckling

Suckling is a term synonymous with breastfeeding, and it denotes the taking in of nourishment at the breast. According to recent ultrasound studies, suckling is a peristaltic or wavelike process such as that occurring in the remaining gastrointestinal tract. In other words, the infant's tongue does not move along the nipple. Normally, an infant has an oral searching reflex in which they open the lips and propel their tongue forward. The infant cups the sides of its tongue around the nipple creating a central trough and then begins to suck by grasping the nipple with the tip of their tongue and pressure from the lower gum. The suckling fat pads in the infant's cheeks help create a vacuum. The tongue moves toward the back of the mouth and milk is moved into the pharynx. There is no actual suction involved. Milk is evacuated from the mother's breast by the combination of positive pressure of the infant's tongue against the areola and nipple (the teat) and augmented intraductal pressure in the mother. The nipple is very elastic and lengthens to accommodate the suckling.

Coordination with swallowing and breathing
A fetus develops the ability to swallow during the second trimester (week 24) of gestation and uses this in utero to swallow amniotic fluid. Therefore the swallowing reflex is already present at birth and ready for breastfeeding. Infant sucking is a component of the swallow. Initially, when the baby is about 4 days old, swallowing and sucking (whether on the breast or via a bottle) are perfectly coordinated. Later, the infant usually sucks at least twice as often as they swallow. The timing of the swallowing has been demonstrated to be the pause between expiration and inspiration. About half of a full-feeding is consumed by the infant within 2 minutes and most is completed by 4 minutes. Sucking patterns are not dependent on fat content but newborns do respond to high carbohydrate levels. Infants fed breast milk, whether by breastfeeding or bottle, are less likely to have breathing problems than those receiving formula or other fluids. Breathing is usually not an issue and occurs at the same rate as suckling and swallowing because newborns are generally nose breathers; infant cyanosis occurs but recovery is swift.

Abnormal suckling patterns
Normal suckling by a newborn placed on the mother's abdomen occurs within the first hour of birth. If the infant does not breastfeed and establish a correct suckling pattern within the first few days, they are significantly less likely to

breastfeed in the following months. One common cause of an abnormal suckling pattern is the use of secobarbital or meperidine during labor; infants exposed to these agents often have low suck rates and pressures for the first few days. For deliveries using epidural anesthesia, there is some evidence that the drug used and duration of anesthesia may affect the suckling pattern. Chloroprocaine, which is quickly metabolized, does not appear to have much effect on neurobehavior and suckling, but the addition of meperidine or use of bupivacaine (which binds to the mother's plasma proteins) does cause more neurological problems in the child. Difficult deliveries, such as those requiring vacuum extraction or cesarean section, generally cause delayed suckling and later breastfeeding difficulties.

Differences between breastfed and bottle-fed infants

Breastfed infants suckle at a higher rate than bottle-fed children; nutritive breastfeeding has a typical rate of 2 suckles per second (faster rates are generally nonnutritive), while bottle-feeding is almost entirely nutritive. Breathing patterns differ between the two, with the inspiration and expiration portions being prolonged for those breastfed versus bottle-fed respectively. The incidence of low oxygen saturation and slow heart rate appears to be lower in breastfed infants. The anatomical changes that occur are different in breast versus bottle-fed infants. For example, grasping a rubber bottle teat requires less extension of the baby's mouth than clasping the mother's nipple. The infant's lips are more relaxed and project outward when breastfeeding but they are drawn together when using a bottle. The mandible is used more in breastfeeding. The tongue forms a groove around the mother's nipple and moves from front to back in peristaltic fashion during nursing, whereas it goes up and forward in bottle-

feeding. A child who uses the bottle makes a high-pitched squeaking noise after inspiration and before beginning another suck, but the breastfed infant is silent, or when older, may coo.

Stooling patterns

Stooling patterns of breastfed infants generally change with length of breastfeeding and bear a relationship to milk intake. In the first few days after breastfeeding, black stools called meconium are expelled. Stools become lighter and green or yellow in color and usually are more frequent, copious, loose, explosive, and sweet in smell during the next few weeks. The most prevalent flora is lactobacilli and bifidobacteria (as opposed to the coli forms and enterococci found in stools of infants receiving formula). At about 6 weeks, stools become more solid due to a shift in the mother's milk ratio of whey to casein from 9:1 to 4:1 (and later almost equal). If any other type of formula or food is ingested, stools will be darker, curdier, smellier, and less frequent. A healthy stool frequency is at least once (usually more) per day during the first month to 6 weeks. Stooling a few times a week after that time period is normal.

Hepatic function in infants

Most newborns experience physiological jaundice. Their bilirubin levels typically begin rising at about 24 hours old and peak during their third or fourth day of life. The spike is especially high in infants of Asian origin. Fortunately, bilirubin levels generally return to normal within the first month and no special precautions are needed. The majority of breastfed infants develop breast milk jaundice toward the end of the first month or during the second month of life. Breast milk jaundice is characterized by bilirubin levels greater than 5 mg/dL. Again this is usually not a cause for alarm and painful blood drawing to test for hyperbilirubinemia is generally not indicated. Prolonged jaundice can generally be relieved through measures ensuring adequate breastfeeding as well as phototherapy, the exposure to sunlight.

Colic

Colic is excessive crying and irritability in an infant, usually as a result of stomach or intestinal pain due to cramping. The infant's cry is very high-pitched. Colic should not be confused with crying out of hunger. Causes of colic related to gastrointestinal issues include hypersensitivity or allergy to cow's milk proteins (either consumed directly or passed via mother's milk), gastroesophageal reflux associated with cow's milk allergy, allergic responses to other foods in the maternal diet, feeding issues like swallowing of air, or smoking. Cow's milk hypersensitivity can be identified or excluded by eliminating all maternal and infant sources of cow's milk and keeping a food and behavior diary. Infant clearance of cow's milk components can take up to several weeks. Although less frequent, colic may also be caused by problems that are not gastrointestinal in nature. Colic may be alleviated through measures such as changing carrying positions (on the back, chest, or prone in the arm), swaddling the child, or administering oral sucrose.

Nutrition and Biochemistry

Caloric intake, milk volumes and storage capacity, and infant growth

The average caloric content of human milk is around 65 kcal/dL. Breastfed infants typically ingest fewer kilocalories as they grow; for example, at 14 days, they ingest about 128 kcal/kg, but by age 5 months they consume a little less than half that amount. All measurements of daily energy expenditure indicate that breastfed infants utilize fewer calories and have a higher percentage of body fat than bottle-fed babies. Nevertheless, mean body weights are similar in the two groups. Milk volumes and rate of synthesis are variable and dependent upon the needs of the infant. After a large spike in volume between days 2 and 4, a volume of about 0.5 L of milk per day is achieved. This volume rises slowly to approximately 0.8 L by the sixth month. Mothers with smaller breasts can produce as much milk as those with larger breasts, but the latter have a larger storage capacity allowing more flexibility in feeding schedules. The milk yield differs between breasts (generally higher in right breasts). Breastfed infants have similar growth rates to bottle- or mixed-fed infants when length and head circumference are compared. Weight measurements are generally lower for breastfed infants.

Fat content

The fat or lipid fraction of human milk provides the infant with essential fatty acids, in particular long-chain polyunsaturated fatty acids (LC-PUFAs), such as docosahexanoic acid (DHA) and arachidonic acid (AA). These LC-PUFAs are linked to greater visual acuity and cognitive ability in breastfed versus formula-fed infants. Breast milk also provides more acetic acid, a short-chain fatty acid, which aids in protection against infection and development of allergies. The types of fats in the maternal diet affect the fatty acid composition of the milk. Cholesterol levels are higher in breast milk than formula, but by adulthood breastfed individuals generally have lower concentrations of cholesterol than their formula-fed peers. Fat content in milk is variable depending on the degree of emptying and tends to spike as more milk is extracted.

Carbohydrates and protein

The major carbohydrate in human breast milk is lactose. Lactose is metabolized by the enzyme lactase in the infant's intestinal tract into the sugars galactose and glucose. Lactose promotes absorption of calcium, magnesium, and manganese. Typical mature breast milk has 7 gm/dL lactose and smaller amounts of other carbohydrates. Mature milk also has an average of 0.9gm/dL of total protein. The major proteins are casein, which increases during the period of lactation, and whey proteins, which peak in early lactation and then decrease. Whey proteins are easily acidified and digested. There are 5 main types of whey proteins found. Three of these play roles in immune defense; those proteins include: immunoglobulins (particularly secretory IgA), the iron-binding protein lactoferrin, and the bacteriolytic protein lysozyme. The other major whey proteins are alpha-lactalbumin, which contains essential amino acids, and serum albumin. Proteins are made up of amino acids, some of which are free and others; essential (must be consumed). Amino acids and nucleotides contain nitrogen, which is crucial for growth.

Fat-soluble vitamins

The fat-soluble vitamins found in human milk are vitamins A, D, E, K, and beta-carotene. Concentrations of fat-soluble vitamins decrease as lactation proceeds. Vitamin A, mostly in the form of retinol, is usually prevalent in human milk; beta-carotene can be converted to vitamin A. Vitamin A is utilized to maintain epithelial structures and promote vision. Vitamin D, which promotes bone development, is not as available in human milk; thus to avoid rickets, breastfed infants need some sun exposure and possibly vitamin D supplements. Vitamin E levels are very high in colostrum but decline as lactation progresses. Vitamin E is an antioxidant which prevents injury to retinal and lung cell membranes; low levels of this vitamin can produce hemolytic anemia in premature babies. Vitamin K is utilized to assemble blood-clotting factors. Since newborns may not have enough vitamin K until they ingest considerable breast milk, they may be susceptible to hemorrhagic disease and might require vitamin K supplements.

Water-soluble vitamins

The water-soluble vitamins found in human milk include thiamine, riboflavin, niacin, folic acid, vitamin B_6, vitamin B_{12}, and vitamin C. Most of the aforementioned vitamin concentrations increase as lactation progresses. The exceptions include vitamin B_{12}, which decreases; vitamin C, which is fairly constant; and folic acid, which is absent in colostrum. Vitamin B_{12} is essential for central nervous system development and normal blood formation. Another B vitamin complexed to protein, folate, or folic acid is also needed for similar reasons and may be supplemented. Vitamin C, like the fat-soluble vitamins A and E, is a scavenger for oxygen radicals and has anti-inflammatory properties.

Minerals

Minerals are inorganic nutritive substances. Minerals and vitamins are considered micronutrients, substances needed in small amounts for growth and development. The minerals found in human milk are sodium, zinc, iron, calcium, magnesium, and several others in very small quantities. Most mineral concentrations in milk spike a few days after delivery then diminish slightly to a fairly steady state. They are utilized in the regulation of various bodily functions and their concentrations are mostly independent of maternal diet. Elevated sodium levels are associated with weaning, mastitis, malnutrition, and dehydration. Zinc levels are much higher in colostrum than mature milk reflecting the mineral's role in growth; low concentrations may occur in the milk of mothers of premature babies, babies with a low birth weight, or in non-breastfed infants with the inherited metabolic disorder acrodermatitis enteropathica. Human milk contains relatively low concentrations of both iron and calcium, but deficiencies are uncommon because both are well absorbed through breastfeeding. Iron and calcium are used to make hemoglobin and bones, respectively. Magnesium levels decrease with lactation progression.

Preterm and full-term milk

Breast milk from a woman who delivers a preterm child is higher in almost all parameters initially and over the course of the first month or so after delivery than the milk produced by mothers of full-term children. The concentrations of energy, or kilocalories, lipid, protein, nitrogen, fatty acids, some micronutrients, immunoglobulins, immune cells, and anti-inflammatory factors are all higher in preterm milk. Elevated micronutrients include calcium, phosphorus, zinc, magnesium, and sodium in preterm milk, but they may still be insufficient to sustain a very low birth weight infant. Lactose levels are an exception; they are slightly lower in preterm than in full-term breast milk.

Human milk banking

Currently there are 10 human milk banks in the United States and one in Canada. They operate under the standards of the Human Milk Banking Association of North America (HMBANA), which adheres to suggested guidelines of testing for HIV and other microorganisms and pasteurization of the milk. Milk banking is common in many European and other countries. In developing countries, the World Health Organization endorses banked milk but still condones milk from a so-called "healthy wet nurse." Banked donor human milk is by definition species-specific eliminating the possibility of graft-versus-host reactions. It is easily digested and therefore ideal for premature babies or infants with digestive or metabolic problems. Most of the important nutrients in human milk are stable enough to survive the pasteurization process and are thus available to promote growth, maturation, and development of infant organ systems. Human donor milk retains immune factors that ward off infection and help to build the immune system.

Donor milk for preterm infants
The Human Milk Banking Association of North America (HMBANA) gives first priority for human donor milk to premature infants who are ill, followed by healthy preterm infants, and then priority is established by various combinations of medical conditions, age, and functionality. If the mother cannot supply enough colostrum initially, immediate feeding with human banked milk is recommended in order to stimulate the infant's gut maturation. Donor milk is at least 6 times as effective in protecting these infants against necrotizing enterocolitis (NEC) versus formula. These babies are usually of low or very low birth weight (LBW, VLBW), have immature digestive systems, and cannot absorb nutrients properly. Therefore, donor milk reserved for premature infants is often matched gestationally and manipulated in terms of nutrient content and availability (such as homogenization). Donor milk can be made available on demand for larger feeding volumes. One controversial issue is the addition to donor milk or separate use of fortifiers to increase different needed nutrients since these fortifiers are generally derived from cow's milk.

Donor selection and screening and milk processing
Most countries do not pay human milk donors. Generally donors are healthy, lactating women who have delivered full-term babies, although there are exceptions (mothers of preterm babies or those who have died). The donors are initially screened by phone, then via a health questionnaire, and lastly, a serum sample is taken to screen for HIV-1 and 2, hepatitis B and C, syphilis, human T-cell leukemia virus (HTLV-1), and other disease markers. Donors are excluded for presence of any of these markers, receiving recent transplants or transfusions, having questionable sexual partners, having tattoos or piercing, using drugs, and other dubious practices. Preferred collection is pumping milk into sterile containers provided by the milk bank. Serial collections are preferred over single ones. Collected milk is usually thawed and pooled at the donor bank and then pasteurized in a constant temperature water bath at 62.5°C for 30 minutes. The milk is then aliquoted and frozen.

Quality control and effects of preparation
Collection can be somewhat standardized through use of uniform, airtight, sterile collection containers and careful

- 26 -

instructions to the donor mother. Storage parameters are outlined and the length of time until pasteurization determines whether room temperature, refrigeration, or freezing is necessary for milk storage. Thawing is done only in a refrigerator or lukewarm water. The pasteurization process (called Holder pasteurization) is quality-controlled at several points. Quality control measures include pooling and mixing the milk, using a control sample to determine optimum storage temperature, chilling milk while waiting for microbial culture results, and acquisition of milk by prescription only. The 62.5°F pasteurization temperature completely destroys HIV and other viruses and bacteria. Some milk components are heat stable and unfazed by the heating; those components include fatty acids and growth factors. Other constituents have various degrees of retention. Notably, anti-microbial activity is in large part retained (one study showed 70% retention of IgA, which is absent in formula).

Nutritional requirements for the mother

The mother's diet has only a modest affect on milk secretion and composition. The RDA, or Recommended Dietary Allowance, of energy intake for a lactating mother is about 500 calories above normal, but many women do not comply with these guidelines and eat much less. Basal metabolic rates increase during pregnancy and continue to be relatively high during lactation. The impact of energy intake below currently recommended levels is still unclear. Fluid intake can be increased somewhat to augment milk production, but essentially the mother should drink to satisfy her own thirst and prevent constipation. Various studies suggest that calcium supplementation is usually not necessary; while breastfeeding may cause some transient bone loss, bone density returns

to normal or higher after weaning. Instances where supplementation may be needed include vegetarian mothers (especially vitamin B_{12}), others who shun dairy-rich (calcium, 600 mg/day) and/or vitamin-D enriched (vitamin D at 5-7.5 μg/day) foods, and those with other nutritional deficiencies (multivitamin with iron).

Weight loss and exercise

During pregnancy, extra fat is stockpiled to provide some of the energy requirements for lactation. Various analyses indicate that breastfeeding women lose more weight than non-breastfeeding mothers. This increased weight loss occurs despite generally less activity. It begins about 2 weeks postpartum and is particularly discernible during the second 6 months after delivery. Mothers generally experience gradual weight loss to eventually return to their previous healthy weight. Many are very conscious about their weight and try to diet. Extreme diet practices can produce deleterious effects on the infant through release of fat-soluble toxic materials into the milk or deficiencies in milk production, and thus, infant weight gain. Generally, however, even modest caloric intake, such as 1500 kcal/day, is sufficient. Safe weight loss can be achieved through intake of about 2200 kcal a day, reducing fat content to a maximum of 25%, and exercising at a moderate level.

Substances passing through milk

There is some evidence that a small percentage of caffeine ingested by the mother may pass into breast milk, but these small amounts do not appear to adversely affect the child's heart rate or ability to sleep. Premature or ill infants may have delayed ability to eliminate the caffeine. Studies have also shown that certain food flavorings (such as vanilla) eaten by the mother are transmitted to milk. This phenomenon is positive because these flavors appear to stimulate infant suckling, which leads to the baby obtaining more milk and having greater receptivity to a variety of foods later. Allergens may also be passed in breast milk; cow's milk and its derivatives are the most prevalently transferred allergens, but others can be transmitted as well.

Nutritional risk factors

Several nutritional risk factors in lactating mothers are related to the probability of poor dietary habits. These factors include a maternal age of less than 17 years, economically deprived mothers, and those who have limited their caloric intake drastically in an effort to lose weight. Other risk factors are associated with either multiple births or a subsequent pregnancy while still breastfeeding, both of which place additional caloric and hydration requirements on the mother. Mothers who weigh less than 85% of their suggested weight, who did not gain enough weight during pregnancy or who experience rapid weight loss during breastfeeding are also at nutritional risk.

Dietary counseling for mothers

Dietary counseling for the lactating mother should include a nutrition questionnaire addressing her nutritional risk. The questionnaire should include queries about the mother's eating patterns, her ability to obtain enough food, her actual food intake, and lifestyle issues that can impact nutrition. Screening questions should include subjects like intake of calcium-rich foods (such as dairy products, fish, and greens), foods that the mother may be excluding (especially vegetarians), fruit and vegetable ingestion, and dietary restriction in weight loss attempts. Other

pertinent questions include exposure to sunlight or ingestion of foods containing vitamin D, ability to get adequate amounts of foods, and whether they smoke, drink, or use drugs. It is also useful to ask the mother about her perception of her weight. Subsequent dietary counseling should focus on positive reinforcement of beneficial practices, identification of areas for improvement, and formulation and implementation of a plan to address deficiencies. A follow-up session should be included.

Calculating energy requirements

Calories and kilocalories are units of energy and energy-producing potential in foods. If energy is not utilized, it is converted to fat and stored. A rapid way to calculate energy requirements for a lactating mother is to convert her recommended (or desired) body weight, in kilograms, to energy needs in terms of activity level and then add 500 kcal to account for lactation. The calculation is as follows:

Step 1: Expression of weight in kilograms = desired weight in pounds/2.2 kg/lb = weight in kilograms

Step 2: Determination of normal energy requirements based on activity level = desired weight in kg x energy expenditure factor (in kcal/kg, body weight/day) = daily energy requirement for non-lactating woman (in kcal/day)

According to the Institute of Medicine, energy expenditure factors for women aged 19 to 50 years, and whose activity levels are very light, light, moderate, heavy, or exceptional should be 30, 35, 37, 44 or 51, respectively. A moderate energy expenditure factor of 37 is often used to estimate activity levels, but the actual activity level of lactating women may be less.

Step 3: Add 500 kcal to account for lactation = normal energy requirements (step 2 above) + 500 kcal = daily kilocalories required for a lactating woman.

Nutritional parameters for mothers

Lactating mothers should consume approximately 50%-55% of their calories in the form of carbohydrates, such as whole grains, fresh fruits, and vegetables. Twenty-five grams of dietary fiber should be consumed, both in soluble and insoluble forms, daily. Current daily recommendations for protein intake are 65 g for the first 6 months of lactation and 62 g during the second 6 months; protein should account for 12%-15% of daily calories. It is important that ingested combinations of protein include all of the 8 essential amino acids; animal protein includes all eight, but vegetarian sources usually do not and must be combined at a single meal. Less than 30% of calories should be consumed as fats. One fat that may be required in supplement form is DHA or docosahexanoic acid, which aids infant brain development. Vitamin supplements, particularly water-soluble vitamins that are not stored and need replenishment such as vitamin B_6, may be recommended. The mother should consume about 1200 mg/day of calcium, regardless of whether the source is ingested food or supplementation.

General diet recommendations

A lactation consultant should encourage lactating mothers to eat a variety of foods, particularly if they are vegetarians. Vegans may need vitamin B_{12} supplementation. A lactating mother's diet should include abundant amounts of vegetables, fruits, and grain products. Fat intake should be monitored to keep cholesterol levels low, which means the diet should be low in fat (especially saturated fat) and cholesterol (<300 mg/day). The diet should also be moderate in terms of the amount of ingested sugars, salt, and sodium (2.4 gm/day recommended). Alcohol should be consumed with restraint or preferably avoided, as it can pass into the breast milk. The nutritional regime should include foods high in calcium, such as dairy products, fish, and dark, green vegetables. It should also include products containing iron, such as meat, poultry, legumes, and iron-enriched grains. Lactating women should also be careful to consume the amount of calories indicated by their activity level.

Variations in breast milk content

On average, human breast milk contains 3.8% fat, with fat content tending to increase as a feeding progresses. The lipid content of breast milk is often dependent on the time of day, generally rising during the morning and decreasing after midday. The protein content, as measured by nitrogen content, and lactose concentrations are relatively low in the mornings when fat levels are high and typically increase in the late afternoon and evening. The mean percentage of lactose in breast milk is 7%. Whey proteins and casein make up about 1% of breast milk. Ash comprises approximately 0.2% of human milk. Human breast milk contains approximately 200 substances, including proteins, vitamins, minerals, fats, and others. Potential milk volume can differ by time of day and is generally highest in the late afternoon and night. Maternal malnutrition tends to lower milk volume while not significantly changing relative content.

Colostrum and transitional milk

Colostrum is the yellowish fluid secreted by the mother from birth to approximately 4 days postpartum. The daily volume of colostrum produced increases from about 50g to 625 g between days 1 and 4. Citrate levels increase in tandem and then level off. Early colostrum is high in total protein, providing approximately 3 g on day 1, relative to later colostrum and breast milk; the early protein content of colostrums reflects it protective immunoglobulin (mainly IgA) content. Most fat and lipid concentrations are low relative to transitional or mature milk, but most other components are more abundant than in mature milk. These components include beta-carotene, which gives colostrum its distinctive color. Colostrum also contains uric acid and another antioxidant related to ascorbic acid; both of which facilitate trapping of oxygen free radicals. Colostrum contains high amounts of vitamins A and E and the carotenoids. During the first week postpartum, the most dramatic increases in milk content are in lactose, glucose, potassium, and a-lactalbumin concentrations and milk volume. Transition to mature milk occurs between 7 days and 2 weeks postpartum and is characterized by decreases in protein and fat-soluble vitamins and increases in fat, lactose, water-soluble proteins, and calories.

Compartmentalization in mature human milk

The vast majority of human milk, approximately 87%, is aqueous. This aqueous, or watery, phase contains the whey proteins, lactose and oligosaccharides, non-protein nitrogen-containing substances like the amino acids, compounds comprising ash, and water-soluble B vitamins and ascorbic acid. There are also cells present, mainly immune cells like macrophages, neutrophils, and lymphocytes, as well as epithelial cells. About 3%-5% of mature human milk is in the form of a lipid or compound suspended in lipids. Additionally, human breast milk contains fat globules, which are made of triacylglycerols or sterol esters. These globules are surrounded by a loose layer called the milk-fat-globule membrane, which is made up of proteins, lipids, minerals, and fat-soluble vitamins. The casein proteins are found in colloidal dispersion.

Effects of diet on lipids

In general, the mother's diet does not significantly affect the total amount of fat in her breast milk, but it can influence the lipid class composition. Cholesterol levels in milk are similar regardless of the amount of cholesterol consumed by the mother. On the other hand, dietary vegetable oil phytosterols do show up in breast milk. The P/S (polyunsaturated to saturated fat ratio) ingested is higher in low-cholesterol diets, which aids calcium and fat absorption. Mothers who consume typical vegetarian or vegan diets produce milk that is high in polyunsaturated fats relative to the milk produced by a woman partaking of a typical Western diet; this milk is also rich in linoleum acid, which can be converted into longer-chain polyunsaturated fats and ultimately used to maintain membrane fluidity, to synthesize prostaglandin, and for development of the child's brain and nervous system.

Effects of fat consumption on infants

Fat consumption by the mother is closely related to brain and nervous system development of the infant. The brain of an infant increases about 3-fold during the first year of life, and its growth is related to the incorporation of long-chain polyunsaturated fatty acids into the phospholipids in the cerebral cortex. The white matter of the brain and spinal cord consists of nerve fibers surrounded by a myelin sheath; messenger RNA specific to myelin is responsive to dietary fat. The essential fatty acids, linoleic and linolenic acids augment the nervous system

- 30 -

development by impeding demyelination. Development of neuronal membranes and retinal photoreceptor cells in the infant is dependent on docosahexanoic acid provided by the diet and synthesized in the liver; much of this occurs in the fetus. Other fats promote functional and biochemical development. For example, omega-3 fatty acids are used to build biological membranes.

Cholesterol levels

Both cholesterol and n-3 fatty acids are vital components of cell membranes and valuable for growth. Infants who breastfeed have higher concentrations of plasma cholesterol than those fed formula, regardless of the formulation. Newborns typically have cholesterol levels in the range of 50-100 mg/dL, distributed equally between low- and high-density lipoproteins (LDL and HDL, respectively). LDLs increase more rapidly in the first few days of life. Cholesterol levels also increase especially in breastfed children. Studies suggest that the higher cholesterol levels in infancy caused by breastfeeding enable the individual to metabolize cholesterol more effectively in later life, which may result in some protective effect against coronary heart disease and atherosclerosis.

N-3 fatty acids

N-3 or omega-3 fatty acids have a carbon-carbon double bond in the n-3 position. They include the nutritionally important polyunsaturated fats a-linolenic acid (ALA), eicosapentaenoic acid (EPA), and docosahexaenoic acid (DHA). Some groups recommend DHA supplementation in pregnant women or addition of the fatty acid to formula because it is associated with retinal development, visual acuity, and cognitive development. EPA, a precursor of DHA, is believed to be important for neuronal development as well. EPA is a member of the eicosanoid group, which includes a number of substances that influence physiological processes. Those substances include prostanoids (like prostaglandin) and leukotrienes, both of which mediate inflammation. Studies indicate improvement of visual acuity in very low birth weight infants with addition of n-3 fatty acids to the diet. Human milk is superior to formulas that have synthetically added DHA or other omega-3 fatty acids.

Protein in human milk, colostrum, and cow's milk

Human breast milk, colostrum, and cow's milk (which is in formula) all have casein, whey proteins, and non-protein nitrogen. The largest component in colostrum includes whey proteins, whereas breast milk proteins are comprised of approximately 40% casein and 60% whey, primarily in the form of lactalbumin. On the other hand, cow's milk protein is primarily composed of casein. The major whey proteins in human colostrum are a-lactalbumin, lactoferrin, and immunoglobulins. The concentrations of the whey proteins and Ig are lower in breast milk. Colostrum contains much more secretory IgA, which prevents viruses and bacteria from penetrating mucosa. Both breast milk and colostrum have low relative levels of the major immunoglobulin IgG. Both colostrum and human milk also contain small amounts of serum albumin and the bacteriolytic enzyme lysozyme. The most prevalent protein by concentration in cow's milk is B-lactoglobulin; a-lactalbumin which contains essential amino acids is much lower and the antimicrobial agent's lactoferrin and lysozyme are only found in trace amounts.

Non-protein nitrogen

Non-protein nitrogen (NPN) is lower in cow's milk (3%-5%) than human milk (18%-30%). Concentrations of many forms of NPN decrease in later human milks. NPN is found in various functional varieties. It is present as the amino sugars N-acetylglucosamine and N-acetylneuraminic acid and various peptides, all of which play roles in development of the gut. These peptides include epidermal growth factor, somatomedin-C, and insulin. Another peptide, delta sleep-inducing peptide, influences sleep and wake patterns. NPN is also present as important free amino acids taurine and glutamic acid, carnitine (used to synthesis brain lipids), growth promoters choline and ethanolamine, polyamines (implicated in transcription, translation, and gut maturation), nucleotides, and, late in the cycle, as nucleic acids.

Taurine and glutamic acid
Taurine and glutamic acid are non-protein nitrogen (NPN) constituents of human milk. Glutamic acid or glutamine is a free amino acid that increases zinc absorption and is an antecedent to brain glutamate. There are high levels of taurine, 2-aminoethanesulfonic acid, in human milk but only trace amounts in cow's milk. Taurine is found conjugated to bile acids in neonates. Bile acids persist in conjugating to taurine in infants who are breastfed, but they primarily combine with glycine in bottle-fed babies. Another function of taurine is cell membrane stabilization, and it has been implicated in other types of functions, such as osmoregulation and calcium control.

Nucleotides and nucleic acids
Nucleotides and nucleic acids are forms of non-protein nitrogen found in human milk. Nucleotides are not present in cow's milk formulas unless supplemented, which some authorities consider

important. Nucleic acids (DNA and RNA), which convey genetic information, can be demonstrated in human milk after 30 days and are hydrolyzed to produce nucleotides. A nucleotide is made up of phosphoric acid bound to a sugar and a pyramidine or purine derivative. Nucleotides appear to be exuded from the mother's mammary gland epithelial cells into the milk. During the course of lactation, the total nucleotide content is consistent but relative amounts of specific nucleotides may change. Initially, cytidine-5'-monophosphate (CMP) and adenosine-5'-monophosphate (AMP) levels are high, but over time they decrease and inosine-5'-monophosphate rises. Functionally, nucleotides are important for immune defense, protein synthesis, and metabolic processes (serving as coenzymes).

Carbohydrates, oligosaccharides, and glycoconjugates

The primary carbohydrate found in human milk is lactose. Carbohydrates are made up of monosaccharides or simple sugars like glucose, and lactose is a disaccharide or compound comprised of the two sugars galactose and glucose. The lactose concentration in human milk increases slightly over the first 4 months of lactation to an average at level of 6.8 gm/dL; cow's milk has less lactose, averaging 4.9 gm/dL. Lactose promotes calcium absorption and serves as a source of galactose for lipids utilized in brain development. Oligosaccharides are chains of linked monosaccharides. Oligosaccharides found in human milk generally have lactose on one end and fucose or sialic acid on the other; they support growth of the gut flora *Lactobacillus bifidus* and thwart adhesion and growth of pathogens. Glycoproteins are proteins that are glycosylated, in other words linked proteins and carbohydrates. Substances in milk fitting into this category are immunoglobulins, mucins, and lactoferrin, all of which are immune protectants.

Mineral content

The mineral content, or ash, of human milk is related to growth and structural development. The principal monovalent ions are potassium, sodium, and chloride, which in totality are inversely related to the lactose concentration. Cow's milk contains higher concentrations of all three of these as well as approximately 3 times the total salt content. In particular, cow's milk consists of almost 4 times as much sodium as human milk, possibly predisposing the formula-fed infant to dehydration or hypertension. Restricting relative intake of maternal sodium can lower its levels in breast milk. The total ash differences affect infant blood urea levels, which are much higher in formula-fed babies. The major divalent ions in milk are calcium, phosphate, magnesium, citrate, and sulfate. The mean ratio of calcium to phosphorus is higher in human breast milk compared to cow's milk, although formula does contain higher concentrations of both. Over the course of lactation, both calcium and phosphorus plasma levels decrease in breast milk. Magnesium, citrate, and sulfur are all higher in cow's milk as well.

Trace elements

Iron and zinc are some of the most important trace elements in milk. Human milk has only about 100 /dL iron, which is less than current dietary recommendations. Nevertheless, the iron in human milk is absorbed at a much higher rate than that in cow's milk or formulas enriched with iron. The incidence of anemia in exclusively breastfed infants is high in preterm infants and those with low prenatal iron stores. Zinc is a trace element utilized as an enzyme activator and structural component of enzymes. Inadequate zinc can cause failure-to-thrive and skin lesions. Zinc intake decreases over time in breastfed infants to levels significantly less than formula-fed children, but the mineral is more bioavailable in human milk; zinc is in low-molecular-weight fractions facilitating absorption in breast milk, whereas it is in high-molecular-weight portions of cow's milk.

Selenium, which is part of the enzyme glutathione peroxidase, aids the breakdown of lipid peroxides; higher levels are exhibited in infants fed breast milk versus formula. Chromium can increase HDL cholesterol levels and influence lipid profiles, manganese activates certain enzymes, molybdenum is an enzyme cofactor, and copper binds to low-molecular-weight proteins and increases their bioavailability. Fluorine, which decreases dental caries, may be insufficient in human milk; it is used to convert hydroxyapatite to fluorapatite thereby reducing acid solubility of the enamel. Fortunately, public drinking water sources generally provide enough fluorine. Iodide levels in breast milk are actually higher than recommendations.

Recommended dietary intake by infants

The mean recommended dietary intakes for most important electrolytes, minerals, and trace elements are typically higher during the second 6 months of life than the first 6 months. For example, suggested sodium intake increases from 11.5 mg/kg to 23 mg/kg. Requirements for most of the major minerals and other trace elements go up slightly; only zinc requirements remain constant (5 mg/day). Supplementation is rarely necessary. Some instances indicating supplementation are chloride in babies with failure-to-thrive, iron in preterm babies exhibiting anemia, and zinc in infants with rashes. Some people feel calcium levels are too low in maternal milk and may require supplementation.

- 33 -

Chromium supplementation might be indicated for low birth weight infants.

pH, osmolarity, and other measurements

Human milk has a slightly higher mean pH than cow's milk, pH 7.1 and 6.8, respectively, but both are in the neutral range. Each type of milk provides similar energy values averaging 65 kcal/dL. Cow and human milks are almost identical in terms of specific gravity. Osmolarity refers to the concentration of solutes or dissolved substances. Cow's milk has a higher osmolarity than human milk. Its concentration is 350 mosmol/kg of water, whereas both human milk and serum have only 286 mosmol/kg. The solutes excreted in urine, known as renal solute load, are significantly less in infants feeding on human milk as opposed to cow's milk.

Fat-soluble vitamin content

The concentration of vitamin A, which is essential for retinal development, is very high in human colostrum; mature human milk has about half the vitamin A of colostrum, and cow's milk has much less. There are various forms of fat- and water-soluble vitamin D, but activity is found only in the fat-soluble fraction. Levels of vitamin D are low in both human milk and cow's milk and a little higher in colostrum, and supplementation is often necessary, especially if the mother does not receive adequate exposure to sunlight. Vitamin E, which comprises a group of related fat-soluble compounds, is vital to various functions including muscle integrity and resistance to red blood cell lysis. Vitamin E levels are quite low in cow's milk but generally adequate in human milk and even higher in colostrum due mainly to the presence of a-tocopherol. Vitamin K, which aids development of clotting factors and prevents hemorrhaging, is often deficient in the newborn; cow's milk has a higher concentration of vitamin K than mature human milk.

Water-soluble vitamin content

In general, the water-soluble vitamin content of human milk is excellent. Vitamin C, an antioxidant that functions in various enzyme and hormonal systems as well as contributes to collagen synthesis, is supplied at a higher rate in colostrum or mature human milk than in cow's milk. Most of the components of the vitamin B complex are more concentrated in cow's milk. The vitamin B complex includes thiamin (B_1), riboflavin (B_2), nicotinamide, pyridoxine (B_6), antithetic acid, folic acid, biotin, and vitamin B_{12}. Most of these are some type of coenzyme. For example, vitamin B_6 is implicated in metabolism of nerve tissue, vitamin B_{12} affects metabolism of folic acid and methylates various amino acids, folate is involved in erythropoiesis, thiamin helps metabolize carbohydrates, and pantothenic acid forms part of coenzyme A. Often vitamin B complex vitamins are supplemented, possibly with a multivitamin. Even though human milk levels are lower, binding capacity may be higher in human milk (for example, vitamin B_{12}) than in cow's milk.

Deficiencies in diet

A lactating woman should consume an additional 500 kcal/day for a total of at least 1800 kcal/day. She should take an additional 400 mg each of calcium and phosphorus and various amounts of other minerals; an exception is iron, which is not lost as much during secretion as during menses. If the woman is unable to drink milk, then additions of 4 ug vitamin B_{12}, 1200 mg calcium, and 400 IU vitamin D are indicated. The mother needs to eat about 12-15 gm more protein daily for conversion to milk protein. Except for vitamin K, which is generally in excess of

- 34 -

recommended daily allowances, other fat-soluble vitamins usually need to be increased. It is generally suggested that intake of all the water-soluble vitamins be augmented as well. These requirements are based on either increased energy needs or less than complete absorption or utilization by the mother.

Vitamin and mineral supplementation in infants

All newborns should be given vitamin K intramuscularly or orally to prevent hemorrhagic problems due to deficiencies in vitamin K-dependent coagulation factors. Infants delivered at term generally do not require any vitamin or mineral supplementation if they are receiving iron-fortified formula. It is recommended that breastfed infants receive 200 IU of vitamin D a day, and they may also need an iron supplement. In either case, iron-fortified cereal is suggested at some point (4 months for formula-fed, 6 months for breastfed), and high-risk infants above age 6 months may require a multivitamin-multimineral supplement.

On the other hand, preterm infants require supplementation regardless of whether they are breast or bottle fed. A multivitamin-multimineral supplement is suggested during the first few weeks of life; it should contain vitamin E and folic acid. Initially, their iron stores should be sufficient but at about 2 months 2 mg/kg/day iron supplementation is advised. Vitamin D is recommended for all preterm infants. Phosphate supplementation may be indicated in breastfed preemies that develop rickets.

Enzymes

Human milk contains over 20 enzymes. Functionally, these enzymes fall into three types: (1) enzymes related to mammary gland function, (2) those that enable digestion in the newborn, known as compensatory digestive enzymes, and (3) ones that promote neonatal development, termed milk enzymes. Digestion is facilitated in the infant by the enzymes found in milk called amylase, bile salt-stimulated lipase (BSSL), various proteases, xanthine oxidase, glutathione peroxidase, and alkaline phosphatase. Mammary amylase is utilized by the infant to digest polysaccharides. BSSL is one of several lipases in human milk; this version hydrolyzes triglycerides when associated with bile salts. Both amylase and BSSL are quite stable long-term and at low pH. A number of proteases promote the breakdown of proteins. Xanthine oxidase is present during early lactation; it is a carrier of iron and molybdenum and enhances the oxidation of purines, pyrimidines, and aldehydes.

There are two enzymes in human milk associated with the biosynthesis of lactose, phosphoglucomutase and lactose synthetase. Enzymes involved with lipid and fat biosynthesis include fatty acid synthetase used to synthesize medium-chain fatty acids and two enzymes, thioesterase and lipoprotein lipase, that are concerned with uptake of circulating triglyceride fatty acids. Antiproteases are involved with the preservation of enzymes and immunoglobulins; prominent examples include a_1-antitrypsin and a_1-antichymotrypsin, which both inhibit inflammatory proteases. Another enzyme called sulfhydryl oxidase stabilizes disulfide bonds in proteins so that they retain structure and function. Some enzymes found in human milk have anti-infective properties. Lysozyme and peroxidase are bactericidal and two lipases (BSSL and lipoprotein lipase) act by releasing free fatty acids with antimicrobial activity. Several other enzymes have anti-inflammatory properties.

- 35 -

Hormones and hormonally active peptides

There are a number of non-peptide hormones found in human milk. The pituitary hormone prolactin is prominent right after childbirth, and it stimulates lactation. Thyroid hormones, especially thyroxine (T_4) and triiodothyronine (T_3), and steroids are transmitted into milk via the circulation. Steroid hormones include cortisol under adrenal influence and the sex hormones progesterone, estrogens, and pregnanediol. Contraceptive substances can end up in human milk. Hormonally active peptides found in human milk include erythropoietin (EPO), which is involved with red blood cell formation, growth factors, and gastrointestinal regulatory peptides. Some of the most important growth factors are epidermal growth factor (EGF), which promotes gut growth and function, insulin, insulin-like growth factor (IGF-1), and transforming growth factor-*a*, which promotes epithelial cell growth. EGF is present in other fluids as well and acts as a mitogen, a substance that promotes cell division.

Prostaglandins and anti-inflammatory agents

Prostaglandins are a group of unsaturated fatty acids (also called prostanoic acids) that perform functions similar to hormones. They are all derived from linoleic acid in the diet and share structural similarity. Prostaglandins E and F are both found in much higher concentrations in human milk than in plasma. Although prostaglandins are present in bovine milk, they are undetectable in cow's milk formulas. Prostaglandins promote gastrointestinal motility, and they preserve integrity of the gastric mucosa. Large amounts of prostaglandin F in human milk can cause infantile diarrhea. Anti-inflammatory agents found in milk include the vitamins A, C, and E, all of which scavenge oxygen radicals. Additional anti-inflammatory agents found in milk include various enzymes and ant proteases several transforming growth factors, and the immune modulator interleukin 10.

Weaning and introduction of solid foods

The World Health Organization and other groups define weaning as the introduction of solids while continuing to breastfeed. In general, many of these groups recommend exclusive breastfeeding for the first 6 months of life. Age 6 months is a good time to introduce solid foods into the diet of breastfed infants. Reasons for solid introduction include exhaustion of the infant's reserved iron stores, which need supplementation starting between 4 and 6 months. The child can produce enough IgA to discourage absorption of food antigens through the intestinal wall that might cause allergies. This is the time when the child is ready to accept new feeding experiences because they have developed a chew and swallow reflex that allows them to accept food from a spoon. Rhythmic biting occurs later, around 7-9 months, irrespective of whether they have developed teeth. Introduction of solids or other types of liquids before age 6 months does not help and may impede development of the child. Flavors that have been ingested in utero in amniotic fluid, such as those found in mother's milk, help the adjustment; therefore, giving the child cereal in mother's milk is a good way to introduce solids.

Changes in milk composition during gradual weaning

During gradual weaning from breastfeeding in fully lactating women, the volume of milk decreases over time. The levels of protein, iron, and sodium tend to increase during that same period, with a prominent spike in the sodium concentration. Lactose and zinc levels decrease during the weaning process. Other nutrients like fat and calcium fluctuate or remain virtually unchanged. Concentrations of immunologically important substances like secretory IgA, lysozyme, and lactoferrin are sustained or rise a bit. Lipase activity decreases in conjunction with the decrease in milk volume. The solids introduced during weaning adequately replace energy levels needed for the infant, which have been found to be lower for breastfed than formula-fed infants.

Guidelines for introducing solid foods

At 6-7 months of age, a breastfed infant can be started on limited amounts of dry cereal, vegetables, fruit, and meat divided between 4 feedings each day. Initial recommendations for iron-enriched baby cereal are ½ tsp in breast milk increasing gradually to 4 Tbsp. Mild, with later introduction of stronger tasting, vegetables can be introduced starting with 1 tsp and increasing to 2 Tbsp. Similarly, about a teaspoon of fruit, such as mashed banana, cooked bland fruits, or diluted unsweetened apple or grape juice can be started, gradually increasing to 3 Tbsp/day. At first, meats should be pureed or milled poultry with later introduction of lean meats; meat should be served in increments of 1 tsp working up to 2 Tbsp/day. Introduction of new foods should occur gradually and carefully.

The breastfed infant being weaned from breast milk to solid foods has typically been introduced to limited amounts of dry cereal, vegetables, fruit, and meat between ages 6-7 months. At 7-9 months of age, the amounts of each can be increased and divided between the recommended 4 feedings a day. The maximum recommended quantities at this time are ½ c dry cereal, ¼-½ c each of fruits and vegetables, and 3 Tbsp of meat. Solid foods may include soft table foods, such as mashed potatoes, peeled fruits, and toast (preferably whole grain or enriched). If weaning has been delayed until this age, strained fruits and vegetables are unnecessary. At 8-12 months of age, infants will typically consume up to a ½ c iron-enriched cereal, a slice of bread, and a maximum of ½ c each fruits and vegetables, per day. Protein substitutes for meat can include mashed, cooked egg yolk, peanut butter, or cooked beans or peas. Table foods may be served in small, cut-up pieces. Foods that entail minimal chewing, such as certain cooked vegetables, tuna, ground meats, or plain yogurt, may also be introduced. Orange juice may be served to infants beginning at 9 months of age.

Cultural food patterns

Cultural food patterns have little effect on the composition of human milk. Severe malnourishment of the mother can lower nutrient content and volume of the milk. Primarily vegetarian diets, consisting of mostly grains, beans, and rice, are consumed in many cultures and in many areas of the world. For the most part, these diets have not demonstrated negative consequences to the infant because these foods are complementary in their supplies of essential amino acids. Certain cultural belief systems either mandate or restrict certain types of food after birth, and many believe hot foods are more easily digested. The lactation consultant needs to be aware of cultural influences on diet. Some cultures use herbs, galactagogues that may have untoward pharmacological effects on the infant.

Impact of cultural patterns on weaning

Weaning can be gradual over a period of months, deliberate (consciously terminated breastfeeding), and/or abrupt (forced ending of breastfeeding). Early weaning can adversely affect infant health. For example, weaning my lead to diarrhea due to the loss of protective antibodies received from the mother's breast milk or may cause the development of kwashiorkor, and critical protein deficiencies in areas of limited food. Some cultures encourage abrupt weaning through unusual and potentially dangerous practices, such as applying substances like pepper or ginger to the breast or completely separating the infant from their mother (in Fiji). Ethnic and cultural believe systems may impact breastfeeding patterns and the introduction of other foods. Some cultures frown upon feeding a child colostrum; many Hispanics believe that burping causes plugged milk ducts; and some Indochinese practice concurrent breast- and formula-feeding.

Appropriate age to wean

Although the recommended age for weaning human infants is about 6 months, there are other methods of determining an appropriate time to wean, and all of these methods suggest much older ages for weaning. Some practices determining an age to wean include:

- Weaning after the infant's weight is 3-4 times his/her birth weight. This method results in average weaning ages of 27 months for boys and 30 months for girls.
- Weaning once the child has reached 1/3 of his/her expected adult weight. This method results in average weaning ages between 4 and 7 years old.
- Weaning until the child has developed proportional to a specified relationship to the adult body size of their cultural group. This method results implies longer breastfeeding for larger-bodied groups with time to

weaning ranging from 2.8-3.7 years.
- Weaning upon dental eruption of permanent molars. This method results in mean weaning age 5.5-6 years old; adult immune parameters are also in place at this time.

Clearly, most mothers and cultures do not wait until these time periods to initiate or continue weaning. Other triggers to weaning include self-sufficiency of the child, in terms of moving around independently, and another pregnancy.

Immunology and Infectious Disease

Protective role of breastfeeding

A newborn infant has an immature immune system. Breast milk provides numerous bioactive and immunomodulatory factors that provide protection against infection and enhance the development of the infant's immune system. Human colostrum and milk contain immunologically specific immunoglobulins, especially secretory IgA, as well as other classes, immunologically specific cells and their products, and other classes of substances that have immune or protective functions including enzymes, carrier proteins, nonspecific factors, and hormones. Some immunoglobulins are passed across the placenta to the child, such as immunoglobin G, but secretory immunoglobin A (sIgA) and secretory immunoglobin M (sIgM), which protect the mucous membranes of the gastrointestinal tract against pathogenic invasion are obtained primarily from colostrum and human milk.

Accessory cellular components

Leukocytes, or white blood cells, are found in human colostrum and milk in a total concentration similar to that in peripheral blood. Unlike blood, however, the predominant leukocyte type in milk is the macrophage that comprises about 90% of the cells. Other leukocytes include polymorphonuclear neutrophils (PMNs), and T- and B-lymphocytes. The total number of cells and their products drops precipitously around months 2 or 3 of lactation. Macrophages are large phagocytic cells that ingest and remove unwanted pathogens and other substances. They have other functions too like erythrocyte adherence, killing of bacteria, and cooperative interactions with lymphocytes. PMNs are leukocytes that stain with neutral dyes and are capable of phagocytes. PMNs are the most prevalent leukocyte type in blood, comprise about half of leukocytes in colostrum, and are much lower in later milk; their presence in breast milk is primarily reactionary to infection and inflammation in the mammary gland. Epithelial cells are also found in milk.

Immunologically specific cells

Human colostrum and milk contain two types of immunologically specific leukocytes, T-lymphocytes and B-lymphocytes. T-lymphocytes are derived from the thymus and are associated with cellular immunity; they constitute 80% of lymphocytes in human milk. T cells found in human milk are evenly divided between ones with surface CD4+ and CD8+ antigens; functionally CD4+ cells are helper and suppressor-inducer cells while CD8+ cells are cytotoxic or non-cytotoxic. B-lymphocytes have surface immunoglobulins and are associated with humoral immunity and secretion of antibodies. The B designation comes from the area of derivation in birds, the bursa of Fabricius. Both T- and B-lymphocytes react against pathogens in the intestinal tract. All lymphoid cells can cross the mucosal barrier, survive low pH, and occupy the GI tract providing protection, but they cannot tolerate some extremes of external milk storage.

Immunoglobulins

Human milk contains all classes of immunoglobulins but the distribution differs from that found in human serum. IgG is the principal immunoglobulin observed in serum, whereas secretory IgA predominates in colostrum and human milk. Both dimeric IgA and pantomimic IgM are at high levels in colostrum. These levels decrease within a few weeks; IgG levels do not decrease. It is postulated that the sIgA is either synthesized via the gut-associated lymphoid tissue (GALT) or bronchus-associated lymphoid tissue (BALT) pathways after maternal exposure and migration to the mammary glands; alternatively it may be manufactured in the mammary alveolar cells. Secretory component (SC), which binds IgA and IgM to the epithelial membrane, is also found in human colostrum and milk. Immunoglobulin classes IgE (associated with allergies) and IgD have also been observed and are probably produced in the mammary glands. IgA antibodies target enteric and respiratory pathogens like *Escherichia coli,* rotavirus, and respiratory syncytial virus.

Human milk proteins including immunoglobulins survive passage through the gastrointestinal tract remarkably well. Secretory IgA can pass through the entire GI tract and still be detected in feces, as can lactoferrin and alpha-1-antitrypsin. Gestational age at birth can affect concentrations of immunoglobulins in human milk; mothers delivering premature babies have relatively lower levels of IgA and higher concentrations of other immunoglobulins. Malnourished mothers may have lower levels of both IgA and IgG. Secretory IgA levels in milk decrease during the course of lactation. Immunoglobulins are relatively heat stable, enabling use of milk banking. sIgA can survive treatment at 56°C for 30 min and Holder pasteurization (HP) of 62.5°C for 30 min, but it is destroyed by boiling. It can also survive short-time (15 min) treatments at either 56°C or 70°C. HP destroys about a third of IgM and IgG. Storage at -20°C can affect relative levels of immunoglobulins.

Antibacterial protection

Antibacterial protection is provided in human milk through antibodies, the bifidus factor, lactoferrin, lactoperoxidases, oligosaccharides, and immunomodulators. The bifidus factor is a carbohydrate present in human colostrum and milk that sustains the growth of *Lactobacillus bifidus*. Lactobacillus is a beneficial probiotic bacterium that stimulates antibody production, encourages phagocytes, and restores the balance of normal flora. Lactoferrin is a carrier protein that binds to iron; it ties up iron needed for growth by pathogens like *Escherichia coli* and *Candida albicans* and promotes proliferation of T- and B-lymphocytes. Lactoperoxidase is an enzyme that works with IgA to kill streptococci. There are a wide variety of oligosaccharides found in human milk; their antibacterial properties stem from their ability to impede antigen attachment to the epithelium of the GI tract. There are also many types of immunomodulators that bind to various sites in the immune cascade and protect against inflammation and infection; these immunomodulators are polypeptides classified as either cytokines or chemokines. Some of these factors are added to formula.

Transmission of infections

Preventing transmission of infection

Microorganisms can be transmitted through bodily fluids, airborne droplets, or contact. While breast milk can contain infectious agents, in most cases breastfeeding can safely continue. There are standard precautions for preventing contact with bodily fluids, mucous membranes, broken skin, secretions, and excretions in the clinical setting. These dictate that the clinician wash their hands prior to and after patient contact, use gloves if they might touch any of the above or contaminated equipment, wear non-sterile gowns, use eye and face protection if splashing might occur, and dispose of protective equipment as biohazards. Breast milk is usually not considered a bodily fluid by the Centers for Disease Control and Protection (CDC). There are particular maternal infections, such as tuberculosis or mumps, which indicate use of airborne precautions as well. These include occupation of a private room equipped with negative air pressure ventilation, use of masks, and possibly respiratory protective equipment to prevent transmission in airborne droplets or dust particles. Contact precautions are suggested for certain infections; they include a private room and constant glove and gown use. Hands should be washed immediately after protective clothing is removed.

Tuberculosis

In pregnant women

A pregnant woman from a high-risk group should take the Mantoux tuberculin skin test (TST) indicating antibodies and exposure to *Mycobacterium tuberculosis* (TB). If the test is positive, a chest radiograph using an abdominal shield should be taken. A normal radiograph can indicate earlier infection, very recent exposure, or risk of progression to TB. If TB tests indicate the presence of the disease, the drug isoniazid is started immediately or after delivery if the infection is older. An abnormal radiograph that shows calcified or fibrotic lesions in the absence of symptoms suggests the initiation of isoniazid after delivery. If the abnormal radiograph indicates active tuberculosis or the woman has symptoms consistent with TB, then smears and cultures are taken to identify the bacterium. Upon indication, multidrug therapy is initiated with isoniazid, rifampin, ethambutol, and, in most cases, pyrazinamide.

Exposure after infant's birth

If the postpartum mother or another member of the infant's household has a positive tuberculin skin test (TST) suggestive of recent conversion or symptoms of TB, they should be separated from the infant and evaluated by physical examination and chest radiograph. Separation is unnecessary if the person is asymptomatic or their conversion is old. If the physical examination or radiography is abnormal and suggestive of active tuberculosis, separation should be continued and the sputum evaluated by smear, culture, and sensitivity testing. If three smears are negative, separation should continue until inhalation therapy is begun for the child. It should be continued if a positive smear is found until there are 3 consecutive negative sputum smears, and the mother (and/or household member) has received 7-14 days of anti-tuberculosis treatment; the infant should also receive inhalation therapy. If the radiograph suggests previous or inactive tuberculosis, risk studies should be done and prophylactic inhalation and pyridoxine therapy initiated but contact with the child and breastfeeding can proceed. None of these scenarios precludes expression of and administration of breast milk to the infant.

Symptoms and diagnostic indicators

Tuberculosis is generally transmitted as an airborne disease that mainly affects the respiratory tract. Symptoms and diagnostic indicators usually include difficulty breathing, fever, cough, tubercles, inflammatory infiltrates, pleural effusions, meningitis, and/or lymphadenopathy. It can extend to involvement in the bone, liver, and spleen. Diagnostic tests include chest radiographs (which can show infiltrates, tubercles, etc.), sputum smears and cultures to identify the organism, and sensitivity testing to identify drug reactivity and resistance. There is also a rarer relevant variation called tuberculous mastitis characterized by a maternal breast mass, axillary lymph node swelling, and sometimes a draining sinus with or without indications in other sites. Tuberculosis organisms should be identified through cultures of the lesion using needle aspiration, biopsy, or surgical removal of a wedge. With mastitis, surgery as well as anti-tuberculosis drugs are indicated and the infant should not be exposed to breast milk until the lesion heals.

Staphylococcal infections

A large percentage of newborns become colonized with staphylococcal infections through direct contact with others. Contact and standard precautions should be taken. The most prevalent species are *Staphylococcus aureus*, and coagulase-negative variants like *S. epidermidis*. *S. aureus* can cause symptoms like enterocolitis, diarrhea, and cellulitis. Currently the greatest concern is transmission of variants that are resistant to the drug methicillin (MRSA). In lactating mothers, *S. aureus* often causes mastitis. It can also cause staphylococcal scalded skin syndrome (SSS) in infants breastfed by a mother with staphylococcal mastitis. With mastitis and SSS in the child, breastfeeding should be delayed until the anti-staphylococcal drugs like oxacillin or erythromycin have been taken for a day. *S. aureus* and other organisms can cause maternal toxic shock syndrome (TSS). TSS is characterized by fever, rash, low blood pressure, desquamation, and multiple organ involvement; it should be treated aggressively with antibiotics as it can be fatal. *S. epidermidis* often infects high-risk babies with long hospitalizations and should be treated with IV therapy.

Streptococcal infections

Streptococci are round pyrogenic bacteria arranged in chains (as opposed to staphylococci that form clusters). They are classified into serological groups, with groups A and B of most interest. The *B*-hemolytic group A streptococcus called *Streptococcus pyogenes* commonly causes skin and throat infections, which can lead to systemic invasion or acute autoimmune symptoms. Group A streptococci (GAS) are associated with a high rate of morbidity (such as the need for amputation) and death if sepsis or other advanced indicators occur. Standard and contact precautions are indicated, but breastfeeding can proceed after a day of drug therapy with penicillin, erythromycin, or cephalosporin. Group B streptococci (GBS) such as *S. agalatiae* can be transmitted in utero, at delivery, or through later contact. Transmission via breast milk is unlikely. GBS infections are associated with maternal urinary tract infections or inflammatory conditions. In infants, they manifest as sepsis, pneumonia, meningitis, or inflammatory conditions.

Management scheme for group B streptococcal disease

If there is an indication that the pregnant woman could be exposed to group B streptococcal (GBS), she should receive intrapartum prophylaxis (IAP) usually with penicillin or a derivative. If the neonate exhibits signs of sepsis, he/she should undergo a complete diagnostic workup, including complete blood count (CBC) with differential and blood cultures and in some cases radiograph and/or lumbar puncture. If the child does not show signs of sepsis, then a more restricted evaluation of CBC, blood culture, and observation should be done if the gestational age of the child was less than 35 weeks or the mother received IAP for only a brief period (~4 hours or less). Further diagnostic tests can be done if sepsis is later suspected. Sepsis indicates empiric drug therapy for the infant. If the neonate does not fall into the high-risk categories described above, the only course of treatment required is observation for 48 hours before allowing discharge. Breastfeeding is allowed after a day of effective therapy.

Bacterial infections with respiratory symptoms

Respiratory symptoms can be caused by bacteria like *Corynebacterium diphtheriae, Bordetella pertussis,* and *Haemophilus influenzae* type B. All of these can be spread via direct contact with respiratory secretions or airborne droplets and appropriate precautions should be taken. *C. diphtheriae* can infect the nasopharyngeal areas, the larynx, and skin, and its toxin can also cause central nervous system or cardiac issues. *B. pertussis* infection is characterized by initial nasal discharge and congestion (called the catarrhal stage), progression to severe whooping cough (the paroxysmal stage), and then the improving convalescent stage. *H. influenzae* type B causes respiratory symptoms like sinusitis and pneumonia but it can also result in more severe systemic signs like sepsis, pericarditis, and shock. It occurs more often in older children because infants are usually protected by passively obtained antibodies from their mother. Antibiotic therapy and infant immunization is suggested for all of these. There is no evidence of transmission through breast milk for these bacteria.

Sexually transmitted diseases

Bacteria associated with sexually transmitted diseases include *Chlamydia* species and *Neisseria gonorrhoeae.* Chlamydia infections can be transferred to the infant during childbirth and primarily cause conjunctivitis or pneumonitis in the child. IgA antibodies specific for *Chlamydia* have been found in colostrum and breast milk of some infected mothers, but the bacterium itself is not believed to be transmitted via breast milk. Chemoprophylaxis for both mother and infant is indicated; the primary agents of treatment are erythromycin or tetracycline. In the mother, *N. gonorrhoeae* can cause a range of pelvic, respiratory, cardiac, and eye problems. The bacterium can be transferred to the infant at delivery or through later contact but almost never through breast milk. Here the mother and child should be separated for at least a day until the mother has received adequate prophylaxis with agents like ceftriaxone or penicillin. The infant may also need to be treated, especially if inflammation of the eye area is present.

Botulism

Botulism, which is caused by the toxin produced from spores of *Clostridium botulinum,* is normally spread through wounds or eating unsuitably preserved foods. It can also cause sudden infant death through multiplication of spores in the gut and release of toxins, which bind at the interface of neurons and muscles to prevent acetylcholine release. This process may cause paralysis. Botulism in infants is usually detected between 1 ½ and 6 months of age and manifests initially as constipation and trouble breathing, swallowing, or sucking. Stool cultures should be taken. There is no evidence of maternal transmission to the child. Breastfed infants are less likely to contract botulism and tend to experience milder symptoms (likely due to the lower pH of their stools relative to formula-fed children). Some foods associated with greater probability of infant botulism are honey and iron supplements.

- 43 -

Unique bacteria associated with maternal and/or infant infections

There is some evidence that brucellosis can be spread via breast milk. This disease, characterized by body aches, sweats, joint pain, and lymphadenitis, is due to *Brucella melitensis* infection. If a woman is infected during pregnancy, she may abort the pregnancy. Mothers with brucellosis should not breastfeed until they have been given chemoprophylaxis for 2-3 days. In some areas of the world, contact transmission of *Mycobacterium leprae* (leprosy) can occur. Leprosy affects the skin, peripheral nerves, and mucous membranes; the mother should be separated from the child except for breastfeeding and drugs, such as rifampin, administered. *Neisseria meningitides* can be spread through respiratory droplets and cause meningitis, rash, disseminated intravascular coagulation (DIC), shock, coma, and possibly death. Breastfeeding can occur after a day of separation while the infected person receives antibiotics like rifampin or ceftriaxone. *Listeria* has been associated with premature and stillborn delivery (as well as spontaneous abortion of the fetus) and flu-like symptoms; it can be transmitted transplacentally but not through breast milk.

Varicella-zoster virus

Varicella-zoster virus (VSV) causes chickenpox and shingles, which present as skin rash and blisters. VSV is extremely transmissible, primarily through respiratory droplets. Pregnant women infected with the virus can have pneumonia and occasionally they abort the fetus, deliver prematurely, or have babies with deformities or nerve damage. If maternal rashes are observed prior to 5 days before delivery, there is usually time for the mother to develop antibodies that are transplacentally transferred to protect the newborn, but if infection is nearer to time of delivery, the infant can be exposed. If the mother develops characteristic lesions around delivery or afterwards, she should be given acyclovir if seriously ill and isolated until no longer infectious. Varicella-zoster immune globulin (VZIG) is usually administered to the baby. Discharge is affected if the mother, siblings at home, or contacts in the maternity ward are exposed to VSV after delivery. VZIG is given to anyone including the neonate without previous exposure as evidenced by a positive antibody titer.

Measles

Measles virus is very communicable. Infection with measles initially presents with symptoms like cough, conjunctivitis, malaise, and/or white spots in the moth and proceeds to a characteristic skin rash within 2 weeks of exposure. Maternal infection can prompt premature delivery. Measles can be transferred to the child across the placenta or through contact with the mother or others. The infant may just get a rash or they may have more critical symptoms like respiratory problems or bacterial superinfection. Immune globulin (IG) is generally given to the neonate, an exposed mother without previous measles history, and others exposed who have not had measles. If there is evidence of infection (initial prodromal symptoms or rash) in the mother antepartum or postpartum, she should either be isolated from the infant until no longer infectious or with the child if they also have measles until stable. Breast milk does not contain measles virus but antibodies to the virus, including sIgA, are present shortly after the rash appears.

Cytomegalovirus infections

Herpesviruses are DNA viruses with a DNA core. Herpesviruses relevant to

- 44 -

maternal and infant infections include cytomegalovirus (CMV), herpes simplex virus types 1 and 2 (HSV-1, HSV-2), Epstein-Barr virus, and human herpesvirus 6 (HHV-6). CMV usually presents as mild infections, but it can cause pneumonitis, hepatitis, or thrombocytopenia in infants or people with immunodeficiencies. CMV can be transmitted to an infant during delivery; this can be inconsequential if the mother also passes protective antibodies but if the timing is such that this does not occur, the infant can develop an infectious syndrome and nervous system abnormalities. CMV can be transmitted through breastfeeding or other types of contact as well, but presence of secretory IgA generally protects against disease progression. Premature or CMV-exonerative infants should not be given CMV-positive milk, but it can be given to full-term babies.

Herpes simplex viruses or human herpesvirus 6

Besides cytomegalovirus, other herpes viruses can be transmitted to infants. Both herpes simplex virus type 1 (HSV-1) and type 2 (HSV-2) can cause abortion, premature delivery, or a characteristic syndrome in the neonate. Infection around the time of delivery is usually severe or lethal. Later infection in infants is generally a result of contact with oral or genital lesions. Mothers are usually given acyclovir or other anti-viral medications and can generally breastfeed unless they have breast lesions if they are careful (hand washing, avoiding contact with lesions, etc.). Human herpesvirus 6 (HHV-6) infections can result in forms of roseola or febrile seizure. Its significance is unclear because most people are infected with it, and at present breastfeeding is not contraindicated. Epstein-Barr virus (EBV) has been associated with mononucleosis, chronic fatigue syndrome, and certain cancers like Burkitt's lymphoma. EBV can be found in the milk

of a large percentage of lactating women, but the significance is equivocal because infants infected with EBV usually are asymptomatic or have very mild symptoms like fever, rash, inflamed nasal passages, cough, or enlarged lymph nodes, liver or spleen.

Viruses transmitted by animals

Several families of viruses are known as arboviruses because they are generally transmitted through arthropods. Collectively, the most common symptoms involve the central nervous system or are associated with hemorrhaging or other systemic involvement. Transmission via breast milk has not been demonstrated. Arenaviruses are single-stranded RNA viruses that can infect humans through rodents probably via direct contact with excretions, secretions, or their suspensions. Some of these viruses cause critical symptoms like hemorrhagic fevers but lack of information pertinent to transmission precludes recommendations for most of these viruses. Dengue viruses are flaviviruses transmitted by mosquitoes that can cause fever with or without hemorrhaging and shock. Transmission of dengue viruses does not occur via milk, but there are reports of transmission around the time of birth. Hemorrhagic fever and shock are relatively common in young children, probably due to presence of IgG antibodies that further enhance the infection. Marburg and Ebola viruses can cause critical hemorrhagic fevers; the vector has not been clearly identified.

Additional common viruses

Rotaviruses can be transmitted through fecal-oral routes or respiratory droplets but not by breast milk. They can cause diarrhea, minimal fevers, dehydration, electrolyte imbalances, and acidosis. Breastfeeding seems to reduce the severity of or postpone the onset of rotavirus-associated symptoms in infants. Infection of infants with rubella virus is relatively uncommon due to passive transmission of protective maternal antibodies. If postnatal rubella does occur, it usually presents as a mild rash, some adenopathy, and minimal short-term fever. Breastfeeding is not restricted because even though rubella virus can be found in some breast milks, there are also IgA antibodies and immune cells. Poliovirus types 1, 2 and 3 infections can cause fetal abortion or paralytic poliomyelitis is a small percentage of cases. Antibodies to these poliovirus types have been documented in breast milk but no studies have specifically searched for the virus. Polio vaccine is widely available and can be given to the pregnant mother if desired.

Tumor viruses

To date no ribonucleic acid (RNA) from tumor viruses has been demonstrated in the milk of women with breast cancer. DNA polymerase, a reverse transcriptase enzyme which uses RNA as a template to produce DNA, from tumor viruses is found in the lactating breast, however. Breast cancer transmission appears to have some genetic component as siblings, mothers, and daughters do have a greater possibility of contracting breast cancer if one has had the disease. No conclusive studies have been done that indicate transmission of breast cancer (even if virus-like particles are observed) through breast milk and breastfeeding. Lactation has been shown to decrease the risk of development of breast cancer in premenopausal women.

Hepatitis

Diagnostic scheme for acute hepatitis
Hepatitis is inflammation of the liver, usually accompanied by jaundice, pain, and fever. There are many viruses, drugs, and conditions that can cause acute hepatitis. In acute cases of hepatitis, the first step is to look for exposure to the major hepatitis viruses A, B, and C (HAV, HBV, and HCV). Laboratory tests for IgM anti-HAV (immunoglobulin M antibodies to HAV) identify HAV infection; a positive HBsAg (Hepatitis B surface antigen) test can pinpoint HBV infection; and a positive anti-HCV (antibody to HCV) assay is diagnostic for acute HCV infection. A positive HBsAg test is usually confirmed by further HBV testing with the IgM anti-HBcAg (IgM antibody to hepatitis B core antigen) assay; if negative, tests are done to look for anti-HD (antibodies to hepatitis D virus) and additional markers for HBV. If all of the initial screening tests are negative, an IgM anti-HBcAg (IgM antibody to hepatitis B core antigen) test is also done; if it is positive, the person has acute HBV, and if negative, then anti-HCV is usually retested and other viruses and sources of hepatitis are investigated.

Diagnostic scheme for chronic hepatitis
The only known causative agents of chronic or long-term viral hepatitis are hepatitis B or C viruses (HBV, HCV). HBV cases can also be superinfected with hepatitis D virus (HDV). Thus, initial screening uses just the HBsAg test for look for HBV surface antigen and the anti-HCV test to identify antibodies to HCV. If either is positive, the individual has chronic hepatitis caused by HBV or HCV, respectively. If both tests are negative, other causes of chronic liver dysfunction, such as hemochromatosis or autoimmune disorders, should be investigated. If the HBsAg test is positive, further testing with other HBV markers is usually done to pinpoint whether the virus is replicating, nonreplicating, superinfected with HDV, or some sort of mutant. If hepatitis B virus is replicating or actively reproducing, HBeAg (hepatitis Be antigen) and HBV-DNA (HBV deoxyribonucleic acid) tests are both positive; these are negative if replication is not occurring. In either of these cases,

- 46 -

an anti-HD assay to identify possible simultaneous infection with hepatitis D virus is performed. HBeAg-/HBV-DNA+ indicates an HBV mutant.

Hepatitis A
Hepatitis A virus (HAV) is an RNA virus of the picornaviridae group. It is generally transmitted between people via the fecal-oral route or in food or water. Infection is usually acute, mild, brief, and often undetectable in infants. Mothers who contract HAV have an increased probability of premature delivery, which can lead to infection in the infant as well. Mothers should be given immune globulin (IG) and HAV vaccine within 2 weeks of contraction to prop up serum antibody concentrations. There is fragmentary evidence that HAV can be transmitted through breast milk. Nevertheless, breastfeeding can proceed if both mother and child have received the IG and HAV vaccine combination.

Hepatitis B
Hepatitis B virus (HBV) is a DNA virus of the hepadnaviridae group. It is generally transmitted via blood or bodily fluids. HBV infections can produce acute symptoms like jaundice or liver inflammation, but their future chronic consequences are the real cause for concern. The latter can include persistent hepatitis, cirrhosis of the liver, and an increased risk of hepatocellular carcinoma. There is a high rate of vertical transmission of HBV to infants during birth in areas where the virus is prevalent such as Japan and Taiwan and to a lesser extent in other areas. The virus is transferred either across the placenta or through contact with bodily fluids. The primary marker for HBV, hepatitis B surface antigen (HBsAg), has been documented in breast milk, but breastfeeding can proceed in HBsAg+ mothers once they receive hepatitis B immune globulin (HBIG) and HBV vaccine. It is recommended that all pregnant females be screened for HBV and that infants born to hepatitis B surface antigen positive mothers be vaccinated with HBV vaccine and receive HBIG. Vaccination is normally done in 3 spaced doses.

Hepatitis C
Hepatitis C virus (HCV) is an RNA-containing Flavivirus. Acute infections with HCV generally produce no or mild symptoms of hepatitis, but the vast majority can trigger later chronic hepatitis, cirrhosis, and the possibility of hepatocellular carcinoma. HCV can be transmitted via transfusion (rare with current screening tests), bodily fluids, and sexual contact. Coinfection with HIV, certain HCV genotypes, active disease, and high viral load can all potentiate the possibility of vertical transmission from mother to infant. The clinician should thoroughly discuss breastfeeding with HCV positive mothers because although the possibility of infection is low, there are no effective vaccines or immunoglobulin preparations to treat HCV and chronicity, if transmitted, is highly probable. The CDC sanctions breastfeeding by HCV+/HIV- mothers, but HCV+/HIV+ mothers can transfer both viruses and higher levels of HCV-RNA via breast milk. Children born to mothers positive for HCV-RNA should be tested for alanine aminotransferase (ALT) levels during the first 15 months and HCV-RNA and anti-HCV around 18-24 months.

Associated viruses
Hepatitis delta virus (HDV) is a defective virus that superinfects individuals infected with HBV and increases acute and chronic hepatic symptoms. Hepatitis E virus (HEV) is an RNA virus of the Caliciviridae group that is spread through the fecal-oral route or contaminated food or water. HEV symptoms are acute, infection can be fatal in pregnant women, and vaccines are not yet available, but there is no indication of transmission

through breast milk. Hepatitis G virus (HGV) is another RNA virus that has not been classified; ongoing, inconclusive studies implicate vertical transmission around the time of delivery but transfer probably does not occur during breastfeeding. TT virus (TTV) is a newly discovered DNA virus; limited data suggest it can be vertically transmitted to the fetus, in breast milk, and post-transfusion.

Additional prominent viruses

There are dozens of types of DNA-containing human papillomaviruses (HPV). They are transmitted via sexual or direct routes. HPV viruses cause genital warts and growths, laryngeal lesions, and cervical cancer (limited to certain types). HPV can be transferred vertically but probably not though breast milk. Human parvovirus B-19 (single stranded DNA) can be vertically transferred causing symptoms like inflammation of the liver and central nervous system, inflamed blood vessels, and anemia. The virus can also be transmitted through direct contact with respiratory droplets and is prevalent in school-aged children. Transmission via breast milk has not been documented.

Human T-cell leukemia viruses

Human T-cell leukemia viruses type I and type II (HTLV-I, HTLV-II) are retroviruses that utilize reverse transcriptase for replication. Both are endemic in Japan, the Caribbean, and in some other areas. HTLV-I primarily causes adult T-cell leukemia/lymphoma (ATL). It is transmitted via sexual contact, blood, breastfeeding, and occasionally in utero or during birth. Breastfeeding should be avoided by HTLV-I positive mothers or other measures to reduce viral load undertaken (such as freezing and thawing breast milk or reducing length of breastfeeding). HTLV-II is transmitted through intravenous drug use, blood,

sexual contact, and, again, breastfeeding, which should be avoided or limited in positive mothers. The main problems associated with HTLV-II are neurologic ataxias, leukemias, and autoimmune disorders.

HIV-1

There is conclusive evidence that the retrovirus human immunodeficiency virus type 1 (HIV-1) can be transmitted in the peripartum period and through breastfeeding in addition to other routes, such as sexual contact or blood contact. HIV-1 with or without associated cellular components has been documented in breast milk. Risk of transfer increases with higher viral load; lower levels of antiviral substances, antibodies or cytotoxic T-lymphocytes in breast milk; or presence of mastitis or breast lesions. In developed countries like the United States where alternatives to breast milk are available, mothers should be advised against breastfeeding. In other areas of the world, various organizations have suggested ways to reduce HIV transmission. These include antiretroviral drugs administered to mother and child, pasteurization of the milk, education, early weaning, exclusive breastfeeding, and supportive treatment. Studies have shown greater transmission with mixed over exclusive breastfeeding. The antigenically-related HIV-2 virus is less likely to be passed vertically or via breast milk.

Viruses associated with respiratory problems

Viruses associated with respiratory problems include respiratory syncytial virus (RSV) and severe acute respiratory syndrome (SARS)-associated corona virus (CoV). RSV is transferred through infected respiratory secretions via droplets or direct contact. Infection presents in infants as congestion, mucous secretions, or apnea. There is no significant evidence of vertical or breast milk transmission. Infants at high risk for infection, such as those in nurseries, are often given RSV immune globulin (RSV-IGIV) as a preventive measure. SARS-CoV is the main virus currently linked to SARS. Little is conclusively known about SARS at present except that it is primarily transmitted via droplets and not via other modes such as breast milk.

Other viruses contracted by mothers or infants

Animals, such as raccoons and bats, carry rabies virus in their saliva and nervous tissues. Rabies can be spread to humans through rabid animal bites or other contact. The central nervous system is affected causing seizures or changes in mental status. There is no indication of vertical or breast milk transfer, but symptomatic mothers are generally separated from their infants. Exposed individuals should receive a rabies vaccine.

Smallpox is caused by the vaccinia virus and presents as fever followed by a characteristic rash. It can be transmitted during the fever stage via droplets or through later contact with the rash. Vertical or breast milk transfer is unlikely. Smallpox vaccination appears to place some people at risk for sequelae and should not coincide with breastfeeding or be administered to infants less than 1 year of age. West Nile virus, which is spread in humans by mosquito bites, can cause fever, rash, meningoencephalitis, paralysis, and death. It can also be transmitted by contact with blood or through transfusion. There is an anecdotal case of breast milk transmission, but currently breastfeeding by infected mothers is not contraindicated.

Spirochetes

Spirochetes are coiled rod-shaped bacteria. The two main diseases associated with spirochetes are Lyme disease and syphilis. The causative agent of syphilis is the spirochete *Treponema pallidum.* Syphilis can be acquired sexually or congenitally by crossing the placenta during pregnancy or birth. Syphilis presents as highly infectious moist lesions or secretions. Transmission via breast milk is unlikely unless lesions are found on the breast or nipple. In the latter case, the mother should receive penicillin therapy before breastfeeding. Lyme disease is caused by *Borrelia burgdorferi* infection carried by ticks. It presents locally in early stages and progresses to disseminated symptoms later. Initially the infected individual may only have symptoms like joint pain, malaise, or headache and the serious neuropathic and cardiac complications are only evident later. Diagnostic tests for Lyme disease are not standardized and little is known regarding breast milk transmission. Ceftriaxone and penicillin are commonly used treatments.

Toxoplasmosis

A parasite is an organism that thrives in association with another, often at the expense of the latter. Most parasites of interest are protozoa (spore-producing sporozoa) that feed on organic material. *Toxoplasma gondii* is a sporozoa that causes toxoplasmosis; cats and occasionally other animals are carriers. Toxoplasmosis usually presents with vague symptoms like fever or rash remit without treatment. However, if congenital toxoplasmosis is acquired by an infant from the mother at birth, the infant can later develop a range of central nervous system problems such as visual anomalies, learning disabilities, hydrocephalus, or seizures. Therefore, pregnant or lactating women should avoid contact with cat feces, and infants congenitally infected should be treated with antibiotics. No current knowledge precludes breastfeeding.

Giardiasis and trichomoniasis

Giardiasis and trichomoniasis are two diseases caused by flagellated protozoa. *Giardia lamblia* infections are generally self-limited to the intestine producing giardiasis are characterized by diarrhea and malabsorption. The disease is often acquired through contaminated feces or water. Lipase activity in breast milk of unaffected mothers has been shown to kill the organism. Breastfeeding by infected mothers is more controversial, primarily because little is known about infant safety related to the drugs used to treat giardiasis; a safe drug is the aminoglycoside paramomycin. *Trichomonas vaginalis* can be transferred sexually causing vaginitis or to an infant via passage through the birth canal (possibly seen after birth as vaginal discharge). Many women of childbearing age are infected with *T. vaginalis* and the presence of estrogens during pregnancy makes treatment tougher. Infant safety associated with the suggested drug metronidazole is unclear. Recommendations regarding infected lactating women are initial topical treatments like povidone-iodine preparations; if metronidazole is needed; expressed breast milk must be discarded for about a day before breastfeeding.

Malaria

Malaria is a parasitic infection that can be transmitted via mosquito bites (usually limited to endemic areas), transfusion, or across the placenta. It is caused by one of 4 species of the sporozoa genus *Plasmodium.* The congenital version is usually transmitted by the species *P. vivax* or *P. falciparum*, and it manifests as fever, anemia, and evidence of spleen or liver problems in the infant. Later infection generally produces more severe symptoms and possibly death and appears to be associated with mosquito bites, not breastfeeding. The usual drug of choice to treat malaria, mefloquine, has not received approval for use in pregnant females or infants; nevertheless, it not found in high concentration in breast milk and is administered to breastfeeding mothers. It is recommended that breastfeeding mothers briefly discard milk before feeding their children. Infants are administered a related drug called primaquine.

Candidiasis

Candidiasis, or yeast infections, can be spread by a number of fungal species of the genus *Candida,* the most prevalent being *C. albicans.* Candida infections are generally transmitted through direct contact, exposure to infected secretions, or transit through the birth canal. They present in women as mild mucocutaneous symptoms, vulvovaginitis, or mastitis; the child normally develops oral thrush (white patches) or diaper rash. Susceptibility is increased with coinfections, impaired resistance (HIV, prematurity, low birth weight, etc.), or damaged mucosa or skin. Mother and child can easily recolonize one another during breastfeeding, which indicates dual treatment. Topical agents such as nystatin are suggested as front-line treatments. If topical therapy is ineffective, systemic treatment with fluconazole is generally initiated. Amphotericin B is often given to infants with very insidious infections in conjunction with fluconazole or other agents. Fungal growth can also be curbed through maternal ingestion of acidophilus to encourage normal bacterial colonization, reduction of sugar intake, and discontinuation of other antibiotics.

Immunization of breastfed infants

Immunizations or vaccinations utilize modified forms of potential pathogens to protect an individual against infection. They are made from either live pathogens that have been attenuated, made less virulent, or synthetic forms, usually recombinant in origin. The idea is to stimulate protective antibody responses to important antigens. It is the position of the American Academy of Pediatricians that standard vaccination schedules should be followed regardless of infant feeding method. This includes vaccination of the child for diphtheria-pertussis-tetanus (DPT), oral poliovirus vaccine (OPV), rubella, mumps, measles, and *Haemophilus influenzae* type B. OPV and rubella vaccines are made with live attenuated virus; the only contraindication of which is that pregnant women should not receive the rubella vaccine. If necessary, a mother may also receive vaccinations during the postpartum period.

Allergies and Food Sensitivities

Atopy

Atopy is an allergic reaction to foreign antigen exposure. It is characterized by symptoms such as asthma, hay fever, or skin reactions such as hives or eczema. It is mediated through an immunoglobulin class called IgE and a type of cell called the mast cell, which releases histamine. The most reliable markers for risk development of atopy in infants are a history of allergic disease in one or both of the parents and cord serum blood levels of total IgE above 100 Units/mL. High levels of maternal IgE have been correlated with infant concentrations and the propensity for development of allergies. Eosinophilia, high numbers of white blood cells that bind the stain eosin, and mast cells may be indicative of atopy. Characterization of lymphocytes may prove important for predictive purposes as well.

Prophylactic measures for reduction
Many prophylactic measures for reduction of atopic disease in infants have been tried. As manipulation of genetic material related to IgE production is not currently feasible, most studies have examined feeding patterns. Successful approaches have included breastfeeding, use of soy milk in formula, and maternal avoidance diets in late pregnancy. In particular, breastfeeding can have a protective effect against development of allergies by two mechanisms: (1) direct abolition of exposure to foreign antigens in nonhuman cow's milk and (2) transfer of maternal secretory IgA (sIgA) antibodies via breast milk to the infant. sIgA is produced in the mother's gut in response to various pathogens and antigens and passed on to affect the processing of similar antigens in the infant's intestine. Breastfeeding has also been found to suppress IgE levels. Reduction of atopy through control of the maternal diet in the third trimester is less clear-cut. Breastfeeding has been loosely associated with long-term reduction in food allergies, respiratory allergies, and eczema in children.

Changes in immunologic parameters related to breastfeeding

Infants fed cow's milk develop hemagglutinating antibodies, primarily of the IgG class, as early as 1 month of age. This process may be averted by breastfeeding and later introduction of cow's milk. Secretory IgA passed through milk not only protects the infant against invading antigens, but it also binds to and aids breakdown and utilization of oligopeptides in the intestinal tract. Breastfed infants do not develop the secretory IgE against bovine proteins. Eosinophilia can be demonstrated in nasal secretions of children with respiratory allergies or those who have been given solid food at an early age. Exposure to bovine milk through formula feeding can definitely increase the risk of eczema and likely increases the risk for other allergic diseases, such as asthma, hay fever, ulcerative colitis, other intestinal diseases, and infections.

Cow's milk allergy

Reactions to cow's milk can produce symptoms like asthma, eczema, urticaria, rhinitis, colic, failure-to-thrive, and sleep problems in infants. Some clinical disease patterns associated with infant formula use can be considered cow's milk allergy. These include (1) food allergy or hypersensitivity associated with immune mechanisms including but not restricted to IgE, and (2) acute hypersensitivity reactions known as food anaphylaxis mediated by IgE antibodies and chemical mediators like histamine. Other reactions have different mechanisms. These include (1) food intolerance in association with some type of enzyme deficiency, (2) idiosyncratic adverse food reactions that are not well-understood, and (3) anaphylactoid reactions that are provoked by mediator release but do not involve the immune system.
<u>Acute reactions in breastfed infants</u>

Babies who have been breastfed or fed soy milk formula can develop acute allergic symptoms such as urinary symptoms, wheezing, or even anaphylactic shock upon introduction of cow's milk. Studies indicate that these adverse reactions result from some sort of prior exposure to cow's milk antigens. This prior exposure can occur in utero, through earlier introduction of small

amounts of cow's milk, unintentional feeds of cow's milk, or via breast milk if the maternal diet includes excessive amounts of dairy. Mothers at high risk for delivering allergic babies should begin elimination diets in which they cut out the most egregious potential allergens, cow's milk and eggs

Value of breastfeeding

Consensus opinions concur that for the general population, exclusive breastfeeding diminishes the risk of developing asthma and atopic dermatitis. Any breastfeeding can decrease the probability of persistent wheezing in association with infection. Breastfeeding is correlated with protective effects for a minimum of the first 4 months of life, and its effects continue to at least age 10. Early exposure to bovine milk is more associated with cow's milk allergy in infancy than later. For children with one or more parents with a history of atopy, breastfeeding is even more beneficial to protect against development of allergic symptoms against cow's milk. In these individuals, the best alternative to breast milk is hydrolyzed (or partially hydrolyzed) cow's milk formula.

Pathology

Factors affecting ability to breastfeed

Cesarean delivery

Cesarean delivery does not affect milk content or production. However, the anesthetic may affect breast-milk production. The epidural block, bupivacaine, is the recommended anesthetic, which does not depress neonatal muscle tone and strength. Morphine is also usually safe, but there are reports of transplacental passage to the infant, which can suppress early suckling responses. Mothers recovering from anesthesia must lie flat and turn to their side to feed in order to avoid a spinal headache. If the infant cannot engage the breast or if the mother is in intensive care, breast milk may be pumped for use. Pain relief medications, such as ibuprofen, acetaminophen, or codeine are recommended during cesarean recovery and should be administered after breastfeeding.

Obstetric complications

The most likely obstetric complications that can affect the ability to breastfeed are toxemia and vascular disorders. Toxemia is the presence of toxic substances in the blood, and it is usually identified by the existence of hypertension and protein in the urine. Toxemia can develop into a serious condition called preeclampsia in late pregnancy and is characterized by additional problems like visual disturbances and edema. Pregnant women with preeclampsia require measures such as bed rest, a dark quiet room, sedation, antihypertensive medications, and salt limitation or diuretics. Toxemia can result in small or premature babies, which, therefore, is likely to cause lag time before breastfeeding. Full-term infants can be breastfed once the mother has been weaned off the phenobarbital used for sedation. Maternal expression of milk is encouraged to start the lactation process even if some must be discarded. Another possible albeit rare complication is unsuccessful onset of lactation associated with retention of the placenta, which resolves once the placenta is removed.

Vascular disorders

The vascular disorders venous thrombosis, in which a blood clot forms inside a vein, and pulmonary embolism, in which there is a clot in the pulmonary artery or associated blood vessels, can be life-threatening to the mother. Immediate and precise diagnosis of venous thrombosis or pulmonary embolism is essential. The ultimate diagnostic test for deep vein thrombosis is contrast venography, radiography of a vein taken after injection of contrast dye. The best test for pulmonary embolism is a pulmonary angiography, which, again, is a form of radiography using an injected radiopaque contrast medium. Alternatively, a perfusion lung scan may be used to test for pulmonary embolism. Vascular disorders require low doses of radiation (usually technetium-99m coupled to albumin or microspheres) but breastfeeding can proceed. When deep vein thrombosis in the leg is suspected, scanning is done with iodine-125 fibrinogen necessitating a 2 week window of milk discard. Treatment for deep vein thrombosis is parenteral administration of the anticoagulant heparin, which cannot pass into breast milk. In some cases administration of warfarin, an agent that can be transmitted via breast milk, may be indicated.

Maternal Conditions

Mastitis

Mastitis is sudden onset, generally unilateral, swelling and redness of the breast caused by an infection. It is distinguished from engorgement or a plugged duct by the presence of fever of at least 101°F, flu-like symptoms, extreme localized pain, cracked or painful nipples, and systemic illness. Engorgement or plugging can predispose a woman to mastitis as can factors like poor ductal drainage or lowered immunity. Major infectious agents associated with mastitis are *Staphylococcus aureus, Escherichia coli*, and sometimes Streptococcal infections. Maternal antibiotic therapy is indicated. Occasionally incision and drainage of the infected area are also necessary. Merely emptying the breast with infectious mastitis is insufficient treatment. Diagnostic tests include leukocyte counts, bacterial counts, and bacterial cultures. Infectious mastitis is characterized by high leukocyte counts ($>10^6$), elevated bacterial counts ($>10^3$), and high salt levels.

Management protocol
The mother should be confined to bed rest and started on antibiotic therapy for 1 ½- 2 weeks. She should start nursing with the unaffected breast, while the affected side subsides and is emptied through pumping. Eventually the woman should nurse with both breasts. The choice of antibiotic depends on the suspected or identified organism, safety issues, and whether the mother is allergic to any drugs. Generally safe broad-spectrum antibiotics are first-generation cephalosporins, dicloxacillin/oxacillin, amoxicillin/clavulanate (for gram-negative organisms), and erythromycin or clindamycin (for women allergic to penicillin or cephalosporins). In order to make the mother as comfortable as possible, warm packs (or sometimes ice packs) are locally applied, and she should be given adequate fluids and mild analgesics like ibuprofen. Her bra should be supportive but not tight.

Recurrent or chronic mastitis
Recurrent or chronic mastitis is due to chronic bacterial infection resulting from inadequate antibiotic therapy, secondary fungal infections, and/or other breast diseases like tumors or cysts. Bacterial infection indicates continued antibiotic treatment including, if necessary, low-dose therapy throughout lactation. Secondary fungal or yeast infections, particularly *Candida albicans*, are common causes of recurrent mastitis. These can be distinguished by the type of pain, which is a burning, throbbing pain along the mammary ducts. Chronic mastitis associated with fungal infection requires treatment of the nipple and areola with nystatin cream after feeding, and oral nystatin should be administered to the child regardless of their symptomatic profile. Oral fluconazole (Diflucan) is an alternative for the mother. If the mother has a concurrent vaginal yeast infection, it should be locally treated as well. Recurrent mastitis caused by cysts or tumors presents as a unilateral immovable lump, as opposed to shifting lumpiness in a normal lactating breast.

Complications and unusual presentations
An abscess is a localized collection of pus, usually in association with inflamed tissue, and is caused by bacterial infection. Abscesses can develop in the breast as a result of inadequate treatment of the underlying infection. If the abscess drains externally and far enough from the nipple/areola area, milk should not contain offending bacteria. However, if it erupts into the ducts, bacteria in milk can infect the breastfeeding infant, who should be treated with antibiotics while breastfeeding is continued using the other

breast. Breast abscesses are usually treated by a combination of surgical drainage; antibiotics, periodic emptying of the breast through suckling or pumping, warm soaking, and rest. Incisions made for drainage usually heal enough to resume breastfeeding within about 4 days. Mastitis, which usually presents unilaterally, can occur bilaterally if the underlying infection is Streptococcus or in some cases of concurrent non-Hodgkin's lymphoma. Granulomatous mastitis is an inflammatory (probably autoimmune) condition also characterized by breast masses and skin sores; it is treated with steroids, and the area is excised.

Galactorrhea

Galactorrhea is inappropriate lactation or the spontaneous flow of milk from the nipple. The term is usually associated with milk flow after the infant is no longer breastfeeding. The primary mechanism of this flow is believed to be augmented prolactin production, but this is unclear because prolactin levels and milk production are not always correlated to galactorrhea. Causes of galactorrhea include pituitary adenomas and thyroid disorders (both hyper- and hypothyroidism), use of certain drugs (mostly those affecting the nervous system or contraceptives), and use of an intrauterine device. Galactorrhea can also occur with concurrent amenorrhea as a result of some of the same causes; in addition, the combination can result from other disorders, such as renal disease, chest lesions, and certain hyperprolactinemic disorders. Women experiencing inappropriate lactation with normal menstruation, fertility, and prolactin levels are said to have idiopathic galactorrhea, which may be due to a prolactin-sensitive breast abnormality or prolactin levels that are intermittent or undetectable by current assays.

Syndromes associated with galactorrhea or lactation failure

There are three syndromes that have been described in which galactorrhea occurs in conjunction with some degree of amenorrhea; those are: Del Castillo's, Chiari-Frommel, and Forbes-Albright syndromes. They are distinguished by timing (only Del Castillo's is not a postpartum event) and association with a pituitary tumor (only found in Forbes-Albright syndrome).

Sheehan's syndrome is a disorder in which there is postpartum lactation failure related to vascular damage of the pituitary. Indications include hypoprolactinemia, amenorrhea, hypothyroidism, diabetes insipidus (excessive quantities of urine), and hair loss in the pubic and armpit regions.

There are rare cases of alactogenesis, the complete inability to lactate; this is probably inherent and characterized by absence of prolactin. Acute lactation failure has been documented during extremely stressful events.

Hyperprolactinemia

Hyperprolactinemia is the presence of abnormally high levels of prolactin in the blood, which may or may not occur in association with galactorrhea. Hyperprolactinemia can have physiologic, pharmacologic, pathologic, or functional origins. The physiologic type is caused by excessive breast manipulation or stressful situations like surgery or blood drawing. There are many pharmacologic triggers for high levels of serum prolactin. For example, there are a number of drug classes that block dopamine receptor binding (such as phenothiazines), inhibit its release (opiates), interfere with its release (*a*-Methyldopa), or deplete its

- 55 -

supply (Reserpine). Oral contraceptives containing estrogen, calcium channel blockers, and tricyclic antidepressants have also been shown to increase prolactin levels. Pathologic causes are numerous. They can include primary hypothyroidism, disorders of the hypothalamus, syndromes involving the pituitary gland, renal failure, and lesions in the chest wall. There can also be unapparent functional causes.

Hypergalactia and hyperactive let-down reflex

Hypergalactia, too much milk production, can begin prepartum and extend postpartum. It generally manifests as continual leakage outside of breastfeeding or other stimulus that persists. Hypergalactia is often caused by pituitary adenomas or benign tumors, and these patients generally have headaches and vision problems. Some cases of hypergalactia do not have identifiable causes and eventually subside. Possible identifiable causes are hyperthyroidism or postpartum thyroiditis. Management usually includes use of a padded bra, oral contraceptives containing low-dose estrogen, and/or administration of dopamine agonists like bromocriptine.

If a mother has an initial gush of milk from the lactating breast and flow from the other breast, she is experiencing a hyperactive let-down reflex. This phenomenon can present problems for the infant, such as chocking, gas, and colic. The mother should either express some milk before feeding the child or use pressure to diminish flow.

Diabetes mellitus

Women with diabetes or insulin-dependent diabetes mellitus (IDDM) are more likely to have babies with inborn malformations and problems at the time of birth, particularly respiratory distress syndrome (RDS) and hypoglycemia. Many mothers with diabetes delay breastfeeding because some of these infants are placed in the neonatal intensive care unit, or the mother does not have enough metabolic stores to feed. Nevertheless, studies have documented that breastfeeding is beneficial to both mother and child. There is evidence that nursing can lower insulin needs or even produce a temporary remission of diabetes, and the mammary gland does contain insulin receptors. Mothers with diabetes usually have depressed serum levels of prolactin, placental lactogen, and parathyroid hormone; high glucose levels in their breast milk; and high levels of lactose in their urine. In addition, studies suggest that IDDM in children of these mothers may be delayed or depressed by breastfeeding.

<u>Dietary requirements</u>
Mothers with diabetes who breastfeed need to consume at least 500 kcal more than normal (in other words at least 2500 kcal) to maintain both her daily maintenance requirements and the energy required for milk synthesis and lactose production. Diet supplements body stores of nutrients. In particular, fat stores acquired during pregnancy are mobilized to manufacture glucose. It is recommended that the lactating mother eat at least 100 g of carbohydrate and 20 g of proteins daily to aid in this mobilization. Mothers with diabetes need to be carefully monitored for blood sugar levels and ketones in the urine and blood. High levels of acetone indicate a diet deficient in calories and carbohydrates. Hypoglycemia can lead to greater epinephrine secretion and insulin shock. There is a delicate balance to control blood sugar levels through diet alone, and less insulin than normal is often the key.

<u>Associated lactation problems</u>
Women with diabetes are predisposed to infections. This makes them more likely

to get mastitis as well. The most common infection experienced by lactating women with diabetes is *Candida albicans*, which is usually acquired vaginally because of the high glucose content in secretions. The Candida can also contaminate the breast area indicating topical use of nystatin for the mother and oral suspensions for the child. Infants born to mothers with diabetes are often hypoglycemic and must be cared for in intensive care, which delays breastfeeding; there is an inverse relationship between the mother's hyperglycemia at delivery and hypoglycemia in the infant at birth. There is also a high incidence of hyperbilirubinemia in infants born to mothers with diabetes, which often necessitates phototherapy. The underlying reason for hyperbilirubinemia is unclear. Other potential problems for the neonate are respiratory distress syndrome and low levels of calcium and magnesium.

Maternal hypothyroidism and hyperthyroidism

Pregnancy and regulation of the thyroid gland are intimately related. It is difficult for a woman with hypothyroidism to remain pregnant unless she receives thyroid treatments. If she does have a child, the treatments should continue, and she should be allowed to breastfeed. Infants born to these mothers should be screened for hypothyroidism via examination of thyroxin (T_4) and thyroid-stimulating hormone (TSH) levels. Women who develop fatigue, protracted blues, or depression after delivery should be tested for thyroid disease prior to receiving any other types of treatment. About 5% of women develop transient postpartum thyroiditis presenting with symptoms of hyperthyroidism like rapid heart rate, weight loss, increased dietary intake, and large milk quantities. Serum levels of thyroid indices are mildly elevated, but at about 6 weeks after

delivery these women tend to revert to hypothyroidism and require open-ended thyroid replacement. Postpartum thyroiditis can mimic Graves' disease in which there are much higher levels of thyroid hormones, more significant thyroid enlargement, and continued hyperthyroidism.

Treatment and breastfeeding with hyperthyroidism

If the woman has postpartum thyroiditis, she is generally initially treated symptomatically with propranolol to slow her heart rate and output. She may temporarily need medications for hyperthyroidism and later thyroid replacement once she becomes hypothyroid. There is usually no contraindication to breastfeeding. People with Graves' disease are usually given propylthiouracil (PTU) in addition to propranolol. PTU treatment during pregnancy is controversial because the drug can cause fetal goiter and hypothyroidism. Levels of maternal PTU in breast milk should be monitored, and the infant should not consume more than 150 mg of PTU daily; other drugs like methimazole or carbimazole may be substituted. Lactating mothers should never receive iodine (for example via radioactive I_{131} treatments) because it has a high affinity for milk. Radiation treatments are generally contraindicated for pregnant and lactating mothers.

Polycystic ovarian syndrome

Polycystic ovarian syndrome (PCOS) or hyperandrogenic anovulation is excessive androgen production resulting in irregular menstruation, infertility due to absence of ovulation, conditions associated with male hormones (such as bodily hair growth and different fat distribution patterns), and often insulin resistance. Most women with PCOS must be treated with the ovulation-inducing drug clomiphene citrate in order to become pregnant. They may also be unable to produce sufficient quantities of milk due to down-regulation of prolactin and estrogen receptors; metoclopramide, galactagogues, like domperidone, and pumping are used to temporarily encourage production. PCOS does not appear to adversely affect the fetus as the placenta changes the androgens into estrogens.

Cystic fibrosis

Cystic fibrosis (CF) is a hereditary glandular disease characterized by thick mucous secretions that block passages in the lung. People with CF have difficulty breathing, are susceptible to respiratory infections, have pancreatic enzyme deficiencies, lose salt through their sweat, and often have a limited lifespan. Nevertheless, it has been documented that women with mild cases of CF can maintain a pregnancy and breastfeed. There is a lack of consensus about recommendations for breastfeeding, which range from sanctioning to proscribing nursing. Many authorities recommend that the mother's health status dictate breastfeeding recommendations. In general, mothers with cystic fibrosis who do breastfeed wean early with the vast majority nursing less than 3 months. Breastfeeding can be beneficial to the infant since the milk contains protective antibodies and enzymes. Breast milk should be periodically checked for sodium, chloride, and fat levels in these mothers.

Breast cancer

The impact of breast cancer on pregnancy and lactation depends on the stage of the carcinoma and the timing of diagnosis. If an early stage carcinoma is detected during the first few months of pregnancy, normal treatment procedures can be followed. The initial 20 weeks of pregnancy are prime time for possible

neoplastic growth due to immune suppression and hormone changes. Neoplasms found later in the pregnancy should be treated with surgery followed by adjuvant treatments after delivery. Women with advanced breast carcinomas should be treated aggressively and instructed not to breastfeed. Breast carcinomas are hard to detect during pregnancy and nursing because there is more water in the breast and staging requires use of radiation. If cancer is found during lactation, the mother should be given drugs to suppress lactation, treatment should be initiated, and the child should be weaned. Women who have had a single mastectomy are generally not encouraged to use the other breast for breastfeeding, but mothers receiving conservative treatments can sometimes successfully nurse. Some mothers can have successful later pregnancies.

Joint and connective tissue disorders

Studies examining the effects of pregnancy and lactation on development or severity of rheumatoid arthritis (RA) in mothers are inconsistent. Various reports have demonstrated increased risk of developing RA after pregnancy (especially the first). Findings regarding the affects of breastfeeding on development and exacerbation of RA are varied and inconclusive. Women with RA who breastfeed must be wary of the affects of her treatment regimen. Medications, such as the immunosuppressant cyclosporine are contraindicated.
High levels of prolactin during pregnancy have been found in patients with several joint and connective tissue disorders, such as rheumatoid arthritis and systemic lupus erythematosis (SLE). Pain is normally controlled with NSAIDs, corticosteroid injections, and disease-

modifying active rheumatic disease (D-MARD) drugs. The D-MARDs are the only drugs that preclude breastfeeding due to toxicity; they include the cytotoxic agent methotrexate, gold salts, and the immunosuppressant azathioprine. Breastfeeding can also prompt inflammatory polyarthritis.

Renal transplants or glomerular disease

If renal function has been reestablished after a woman has received a renal transplant, she can usually carry a pregnancy safely and successfully. Transplantation procedures require use of immunosuppressant drugs, and the best maintenance choices are azathioprine paired with prednisone or methylprednisolone. If a mother is taking cyclosporine, she should not nurse. Renal or glomerular disease diagnosed during pregnancy is not affected by the pregnancy. However, hypertension is often a complicating factor with renal disease and must be carefully controlled during pregnancy and lactation with diuretics. Pregnant mothers with hypertension often deliver prematurely or have statistically small babies. The choice to nurse should depend on how well the disease is controlled and the drug choice. High-dose thiazides, for example, can curb lactation, while low-dose diuretics or the beta blocker propranolol are much safer. A women with a serum creatine of > 3 mg/dL and urea nitrogen of >300 mg/dL is unlikely to become pregnant.

Epilepsy and other neuropathies

The greatest danger during pregnancy experienced by a mother with epilepsy is the possibility of seizure. Antiepileptic drugs (AEDs) have varying degrees of sedating effects, plasma half-lives, volume distributions, and binding capacities, which can affect the fetal and infant concentrations at birth. For example, phenobarbital and diazepam both have very long half-lives. Breastfeeding may initially be difficult because the sedating qualities of these drugs diminish the infant's ability to suckle. Nevertheless, at least partial breastfeeding is encouraged because it serves to eliminate effects of the mother's medication on the infant and suppresses the withdrawal syndrome in the infant. Infant withdrawal syndrome can include symptoms such as extreme irritability, shaking, hyperventilation, poor sucking, vomiting, and sleep problems.

Carpal tunnel syndrome, compression of a nerve in the wrist causing wrist pain, has been reported in pregnancy and postpartum. Numbness and tingling in the arms during the engorgement period of lactation has also been described.

Raynaud's phenomenon

Raynaud's phenomenon is a vascular disorder in which there are spasms of arteries, usually brought on by cold. Raynaud's phenomenon usually affects appendages like fingers and toes, but it can also manifest in the nipples as extreme blanching or other color changes and devastating pain. Lactating women with Raynaud's phenomenon need to be treated before they are comfortable enough to breastfeed. The standard treatment is administration of the antihypertensive calcium-channel blocker nifedipine, which may pass to the milk but has been deemed safe enough to permit nursing. Warm clothes and room temperature environments also mediate symptoms. Raynaud's phenomenon has also been successfully treated with angiotensin-converting enzyme (ACE) inhibitors and prostaglandins.

Smoking

Mothers who smoke heavily tend to deliver low birth weight infants. Insofar as breastfeeding is concerned, nicotine suppresses the let-down reflex, and smoking has been correlated with poor milk volumes. Nicotine and its primary metabolite cotinine can be found the mother's plasma, urine, and especially breast milk. Prolactin concentrations are depressed in smoking mothers and levels of somatostatin, which inhibits prolactin release, are increased. The measurable reported effects of maternal smoking on infants include increased amounts of both nicotine and cotinine in the urine, low growth rates, greater incidence of respiratory illnesses, increased probability of colic, and greater rates of sudden infant death syndrome (SIDS). Passive smoke exposure can produce some of these untoward effects as well. Even nicotine removal therapies, like nicotine gum or nicotine transdermal systems, still release nicotine into the plasma and breast milk. Effects of another approach, use of the antidepressant bupropion, are unclear. Mothers who use marijuana expose their child to possible long-term developmental defects.

Nipple discharge

Spontaneous nipple discharges unrelated to lactation are usually caused by benign lesions or malignancies. They are distinguished from secretions, which can be extracted from the mammary ducts. If the discharge is milky in appearance, it is usually classified as galactorrhea. Sticky, multicolored discharges usually result from nipple manipulation, contain only normal skin flora, and can be treated with cleansing; the most common manifestation is called duct ectasis or comedomastitis, which is caused by lipid accrual and ensuing inflammation. Purulent discharges indicate mastitis and should be addressed with antibiotics.

Serosanguineous (pink) or sanguineous (bloody) discharges commonly occur during pregnancy and lactation due to vascular engorgement or trauma to the breast, but they can also indicate presence of an intraductal papilloma. Discharges can also be watery or serous (yellow).

The color of the nipple discharge and the presence or absence of a mass can provide clues as to the underlying cause of discharge, but further tests are needed to pinpoint the source of the discharge. During pregnancy, lactation, and especially if there is nipple discharge or suspected lesions, breast cytologic examinations are done using tissue obtained through needle aspiration biopsy. Normally, cytological examination shows increased cellularity in late phases of pregnancy and variable profiles postpartum, as well as large counts of ductal epithelial cells during pregnancy and lactation. Hyperplasia, increased numbers of cells in an area, and possibly cancer can be identified by cytologic examinations. Lumps in the breast are usually caused by plugging of a duct or mastitis, but continued presence can indicate presence of benign cysts (or lipomas) or breast cancer. Imaging techniques and galactography (radiography of the breast after injection of radiopaque contrast material) are used for further diagnosis. Pain and tenderness can also be caused by benign hormonally-controlled fibrocystic disease.

Gigantomastia

Gigantomastia of pregnancy is an uncommon condition in which there is considerable hypertrophy of the breast during pregnancy. The breast enlargement begins early during the pregnancy, continues during it (sometimes up to 3 times normal size), and then retreats in the weeks after delivery. The breasts are firm and swollen

- 60 -

and veins are obvious. The woman often develops infections, necrosis, and hemorrhaging in the breast and has difficulty performing activities of daily life because of the burden. Women experiencing gigantomastia of pregnancy usually develop the condition with subsequent pregnancies as well; reduction mammoplasty with preservation of nipple and ducts is a good surgical choice for these women. Other types of surgery are sometimes indicated during the pregnancy to address necrosis and bleeding. The cause(s) of this situation are unclear, but it is generally believed to have some hormonal component.

Augmentation and reduction mammoplasties

Mammoplasty is the surgical alteration of the size or shape of a woman's breast. Sensation can be depressed in the nipple and areola areas for 6 months or more. Augmentation mammoplasty is the enlargement of the breast by embedding some sort of inert material in the breast. Since the incision and insertion is near the chest wall behind relevant breast structures and conduits, the woman can breastfeed later. The safest and currently recommended type of implant is a saline gel implant. The Food and Drug Administration now restricts use of silicone gels to clinical trials. In the past, silicone gels, silicone injections, and polyurethane implants were used, but each has untoward complications like fibrosis and damage to the ducts. Reduction mammoplasty to minimize breast size can affect the ability to breastfeed because it usually disrupts the ducts during reconstruction of the nipple. Successful later lactation depends on surgical preservation of both the ducts to provide milk and the nerves in the area to provoke the let-down response.

Dermatitis in the breast area

Dermatitis, inflammation of the skin sometimes accompanied by lesions, can have bacterial, viral, or contact origins. Breast dermatitis of bacterial origin should be aggressively treated topically and systemically with antibiotics for at least 24 hours before breastfeeding. Young infants should be treated if they develop the dermatitis. Viral dermatitis of the breast is usually caused by either herpes simplex or herpes zoster, and breastfeeding should cease until the dermatitis clears. The only exception would be that if the lesions are found on only one breast, the woman can use the other breast to feed. There are several types of possible contact dermatitis. These include latex allergy dermatitis, mastocytosis (hives due to local mast cells), herpes gestationis (related to placenta exposure), PUPP syndrome (pruritic urticarial papules and plaques of pregnancy), and poison ivy. The only temporary contraindications for breastfeeding are poison ivy (Rhus infection and toxin) or any situation that interferes with healing of the breast. Most contact dermatitis is not contagious and is treated with corticosteroids, either topical ointments or systemic preparations.

Pregnancy and lactation and headaches or other symptoms

Women who tend to experience migraine headaches may have worse cases of these headaches during pregnancy. Lactational headaches generally occur between days 3 and 6 postpartum. Prolactin levels are increased during both lactation and migraine episodes, suggesting a possible similarity between the two types of headaches. The connection between lactation headaches and oxytocin levels has not been established, but oxytocin is associated with benign orgasmic cephalgia or headaches during sexual intercourse. There have been reports of anaphylaxis or local urticaria during the let-down reflex; these seem to be responsive to antihistamine treatment. It has also been documented that women with multiple sclerosis (MS) have increased incidence of exacerbations of the disease postpartum. The relationship to breastfeeding is unclear and nursing is still encouraged; the drug of choice for MS is glatiramer, which does not pass into the breast milk.

Conditions in Infants

Perinatal infant problems

A number of problems can occur in postmature infants, babies who remained in utero past the full vitality of the placenta. These infants have generally lost weight, subcutaneous fat, and stored glycogen predisposing them to hypoglycemia (which may necessitate intravenous infusion), low calcium levels, and initial difficulties suckling. During birth, intrauterine hypoxia or inadequate oxygen supply can cause infant asphyxiation due to insufficient placental reserve, umbilical cord mishaps, or other events. The infant's intestinal tract has also been deprived of oxygen decreasing its motility and hormone levels. This may lead to difficulty sucking. Therefore, the newborn must initially receive IV fluids with gradual introduction of breastfeeding. Unique tactics to facilitate suckling may be needed such as use of the so-called "dancer hold," which employs cupping of the breast, or utilization of seats or sling carriers to hold the baby while freeing both hands for support.

Premature infants are not yet able to self-regulate milk flow during feeding; thus, breastfeeding may decrease their breathing frequency and ventilatory capacity.

Gastrointestinal diseases

Gastrointestinal diseases are less likely to occur in full-term infants if they are breastfed. Colitis usually presents with severe bloody diarrhea. Severe enterocolitis is rare in exclusively breastfed infants, which indicates that it is an infant metabolic disorder and/or there is a protective reaction to a component of the mother's milk. Colitis is provoked by exposure to cow's milk, other dietary protein antigens, or, rarely, antibiotics, and it can usually be resolved through exclusion of the offender. Additional therapeutic measures include feeding banked human milk and maternal use of pancreatic enzymes.

Lactose intolerance, caused by low levels of the lactase enzyme, can cause indigestion and other gastrointestinal symptoms. Lactase activity generally declines after weaning. Lactose intolerance can be inherited or temporarily found in premature babies or after bouts of diarrhea. For remission of symptoms, lactose must be removed from the diet; this is usually accomplished through the use of banked milk that has been hydrolyzed with lactase. Possible chronic gastrointestinal diseases are celiac disease, an immunologic response to wheat gluten; Crohn's disease; and other inflammatory bowel diseases presenting in later life. Breastfeeding may protect against these diseases.

Value of breastfeeding for respiratory infections or otitis media

Breastfeeding is beneficial in infants who have respiratory or ear infections. Breast milk and colostrum both provide protection against infection through the presence of immunoglobulin A (IgA). Breastfed infants reap the additional protective effects of IgA in their own nasal secretions. Immune protective factors such as neutralizing inhibitors, IgG antibodies, and lymphocytes specific to one of the most frequent respiratory infections, respiratory syncytial virus, have been demonstrated in most human milk. Nursing infants have less severe respiratory infections, and they are able to maintain more regular respiratory patterns than those who are bottle fed. Otitis media, inflammation of the middle ear, is a complication of upper respiratory infection. Breastfed infants have a lower incidence of otitis media.

Metabolic diseases

Many metabolic diseases are due to inborn metabolic errors related to essential amino acids. Infections, especially *Escherichia coli* bacteria, are often associated with exacerbation or discovery of these metabolic problems. The metabolic disorders generally screened for are galactosemia, phenylketonuria (PKU), hypothyroidism, and cystic fibrosis.

Galactosemia, a disorder related to lactose intolerance (discussed elsewhere), is the inability to metabolize galactose as a result of a deficiency in galactose-1-phosphate uridyltransferase. Galactosemia presents as jaundice, gastrointestinal disturbances, cerebral problems, and electrolyte imbalances; treatment for galactosemia includes weaning to a lactose-free diet.

In PKU, the amino acid phenylalanine builds up due to a hereditary lack of converting enzyme. Phenylketonuria is usually managed using commercially-available phenylalanine-free formulas (usually in conjunction with breastfeeding). Untreated PKU is associated with development of thrush,

developmental disorders, seizures, and tumors.

Cystic fibrosis

Cystic fibrosis (CF) is a hereditary metabolic disorder related to a pancreatic enzyme deficiency. It can present as failure-to-thrive, thick mucous secretions in the respiratory tract, and/or meconium plugs. Breastfeeding is beneficial to infants with CF because it aids digestion and absorption of nutrients and protects against infection. Pancreatic enzymes ingested by the mother or added to formula or use of hydrolyzed formula can improve symptoms and encourage weight gain in infants with CF. Unfortunately, none of the aforementioned combinations have proven universally effective. Mothers are often forced to wean the infant, despite the advantages of breastfeeding, due to malnutrition or stool abnormalities. Most mothers with CF wean by the time the infant is 6 months old.

Hereditary metabolic disorders

Hereditary metabolic disorders that can affect infants include:
- Cystic fibrosis - Discussed elsewhere.
- Alpha-1-antitypsin deficiency - Deficiency of serum protease. M variant is associated with greater risk of development of liver disease in infants and, later, cirrhosis of the liver, emphysema, and mortality.
- Glycogen storage disease type II (also known as Pompe disease and acid maltase deficiency) – Congenital defect related to lack of acid alpha-glucosidase, which converts glycogen to glucose; predisposes the infant to infection, feeding problems, and liver disease.

- 63 -

- Ornithine transcar amylase deficiency - Lack of urea cycle enzyme resulting in accumulation of ammonia in the blood; can cause feeding problems, seizures, respiratory distress and coma. Therapy includes limitation of nitrogen (protein) intake and use of phenylbutyrate.
- Tyrosinemia type I - Buildup of tyrosine and its metabolic products in the liver leading to liver failure if untreated; controlled by diet low in protein, tyrosine, and phenylalanine.
- Galactosemia, phenylketonuria, and other inborn errors of metabolism - Discussed elsewhere.

Breastfeeding is almost universally beneficial to infants presenting with metabolic disorders.

Hereditary syndromes and breastfeeding

Down syndrome, in which the individual has an extra 21st chromosome, is associated with distinctive features and neurological impairments including some degree of mental retardation. Infants who inherit Down syndrome often have difficulty learning how to suck during breastfeeding. The mother may have to modify her breastfeeding technique or use manual means of expression or pumping in order to ensure adequate prolactin response. Some infants may require tube feeding. Breastfeeding, if possible, is encouraged because these infants are predisposed to infections. Down syndrome is also associated with low birth weight, poor weight gain, cardiac damage, hyperbilirubinemia, and jaundice.

Danbolt-Closs syndrome, or acrodermatitis enteropathica, is a relatively uncommon autosomal recessive malady. It presents as a symmetrical rash near the mouth, genitalia, or extremities and has other symptoms like failure-to-thrive and diarrhea. The syndrome is related to a zinc deficiency, lack of absorption of zinc unless complexed to prostaglandin, and weaning. It is treated with oral zinc sulfate and gluconate.

Neonatal breast swelling, nipple discharge, and mastitis

Neonates often have swelling of their breasts unrelated to whether or not they breastfeed. Milk resembling adult makeup called witch's milk can be extracted from the breast. There have been isolated reports of bloody nipple discharges and galactorrhea in infants. Mastitis or breast inflammation is rare in newborns, and most cases are related to breast manipulation in attempts to extract witch's milk. Neonatal mastitis unrelated to maternal disease was more common in the mid-1900s when the rate of staphylococcal infections in nurseries was high, and the incidence was higher in bottle-fed babies.

Bilirubin

Bilirubin is a yellowish bile pigment and cellular toxin. It is a breakdown product of hemoglobin metabolism utilizing the reticuloendothelial system (RES) especially in the liver. Once bilirubin is released into the bloodstream, it binds to albumin (indirect bilirubin), but this binding is less efficient in neonates than in adults. Direct bilirubin is the portion conjugated to glucuronic acid in the liver, which is normally excreted through bile into the stools, and unconjugated bilirubin is in the serum free to travel to other sites. Too much bilirubin or hyperbilirubinemia can cause necrosis of cells and jaundice. In the newborn, cellular necrosis due to excessive bilirubin accumulation can also result in potentially fatal kernicterus or bilirubin encephalopathy of the brain. Infants who survive kernicterus are still at risk for brain damage and associated defects like spasticity or mental retardation.

Hyperbilirubinemia

Many newborns are visibly jaundiced shortly after birth, and standard practice is to monitor serum bilirubin levels. This jaundice can be due to increased breakdown of red blood cells, depressed conjugation of bilirubin to glucuronic acid, and reduced binding of bilirubin to albumin, or greater reabsorption from the gastrointestinal tract. The exact cause of jaundice or hyperbilirubinemia is usually hard to pinpoint, but the American Academy of Pediatrics does have guidelines for treatment. Visible jaundice during the first 24 hours of life warrants evaluation. Acceptable total serum bilirubin (TSB) levels rise in the first few days of birth. Phototherapy or light treatment is considered or instituted on day 2 of life if the TSB is equal to or greater than 12 mg/dL or 15 mg/dL, respectively. Phototherapy is considered on day 3 if TSB levels are equal t or greater than 15 mg/dL and 18 mg/dL, respectively, and for an older neonate, if TSB levels are equal to or greater than 17mg/dL and 20 mg/dL, respectively. Successful phototherapy is defined as a decrease in TSB levels of 1-2 mg/dL in the first 4-6 hours with subsequent continued decline. If phototherapy fails and/or the TSB levels are higher, then exchange transfusion is instituted alone or in conjunction with phototherapy when there is extreme hyperbilirubinemia.

Breastfeeding newborns can develop different patterns of early and late jaundice. Jaundice associated with early breast milk can begin 2-5 days after delivery and only lasts about a week and a half; it is characterized by relatively low bilirubin levels (up to 15 mg/dL), delayed and infrequent stools, and decreased caloric intake. Breastfeeding probably does not cause this condition as bottle-fed infants can experience it as well. Early jaundice appears to be exacerbated by feeding the child water or dextrose supplements. Little to no phototherapy is needed to treat early jaundice.

Late-onset jaundice in breastfed infants occurs around days 5-10 and usually continues more than a month. It is unrelated to caloric intake (milk is abundant at this point) or stooling (which is normal). Here the hyperbilirubinemia is more pronounced, generally greater than 20 mg/dL. In this case, treatments like phototherapy and possibly exchange transfusion are indicated, and breast feeding should be discontinued until tests determine the serum bilirubin levels and the effects of breastfeeding.

Suggested management scheme: All infants should be observed for initial stooling, which should be stimulated if it does not occur within 24 hours. Breastfeeding should be started early using frequent, short feedings. Water, dextrose solutions, and formula should not be added. Weight, voiding, and stooling patterns should be monitored in relationship to the breastfeeding pattern. If total serum bilirubin levels move toward 15 mg/dL, extra efforts to suppress TSB levels should be instituted. These efforts may include stimulation of stooling and breast milk production (via pumping) as well as more frequent feeding; phototherapy is started if the bilirubin concentrations go beyond 20 mg/dL. Transient cessation of breastfeeding is not indicated unless the infant has been jaundiced for at least a week, the TSB is very high (> 20 mg/dL), or the mother had a previous child with jaundice.

Anatomical and neural disorders affecting ability to suckle

Anatomical deviations of the mouth and neurodevelopmental disorders can affect an infant's ability to suckle. Most dictate maternal adjustment of feeding position or technique. Examples of deviations and disorders include:

- Macroglossia - Large tongue relative to oral cavity. Gagging is less likely if the infant brings his/her tongue forward.
- Variations in the roof of the mouth (palate) - Mother nursing in the supine position helps the infant's tongue fall down and forward.
- Atypical oral motor patterns – Characteristic of preemies or infants asphyxiated during birth. These patterns are usually characterized by abnormal muscle tone and require adjustments based on particular abnormal pattern.
- Oral tactile hypersensitivity – Disorder usually develops after use of feeding tubes and can manifest as rejection of feeding, dribbling, or poor suckling.
- Persistent feeding difficulties – These difficulties may indicate a neurodevelopment disorder requiring neuromotor testing.
- First-arch disorders, cleft lip, and cleft palate - Usually require surgery. Further discussed elsewhere.

Oral/facial anatomical abnormalities

The following oral/facial anatomical abnormalities indicate surgical intervention in infants:

- First-arch disorders, cleft lip, or cleft palate in the neonate make feeding difficult and are generally addressed surgically.

- A receding chin is a first-arch disorder. It may be found in conjunction with a cleft palate. Although this configuration makes breastfeeding difficult, it may be possible if the infant's jaw is pulled forward.
- A cleft lip is a divided upper lip. With cleft lip alone, the two parts are usually joined surgically fairly quickly after birth. Before the surgery, the child may be able to breastfeed with help from the mother to create a seal around her areola or with use of a specialized breast shield.

Cleft palate is a gap along the midline of the roof of the mouth and is often found in association with a cleft lip. An orthopedic device closing the gap is used initially and followed by later surgical repair. The ability of the child to feed before the repair depends on his/her ability to make mechanical movements and the generation of negative pressure in their mouth through creation of a seal. Neonates with both cleft lip and palate cannot create this negative pressure; thus, the combination generally precludes breastfeeding. Infants with only cleft palate or a cleft in the soft palate can establish the seal and breastfeed.

Feeding and other issues
The two situations in which breastfeeding is unlikely are combination cleft lip/palate and a cleft palate variation called Pierre Robin malformation sequence in which the child cannot make mechanical movements. Both of these defects usually require direct delivery of milk into the infant's mouth by a cup or syringe. With cleft lip alone, the position of or technique used for breastfeeding can influence success. A useful breastfeeding position is placing the child on the mother's leg facing her, while the mother tilts back and the infant leans forward

creating a proper alignment of structures for suckling. The dancer hold, in which the mother cups her breast and holds the infant in position, is also effective in some of these conditions. Artificial nipples with openings may be successfully utilized with cleft lip or palate alone. It is important to stress to the parents that these oral anatomical problems can be surgically corrected.

Tracheoesophageal fistula and other conditions

Tracheoesophageal fistula is a critical gastrointestinal tract disorder that must be quickly corrected surgically. The baby has signs of GI tract obstruction and respiratory problems, possibly including pneumonia. Surgery to correct the fistula is done immediately if the child has not breastfed or aspirated milk or after they have recovered from pneumonia if present. After surgery, the infant generally has an inserted gastrostomy tube through which feedings of breast milk, IV fluids, and if needed, other nutrient supplementation can be delivered. Eventually the infant can be breastfed or fed by cup. The mother generally manually expresses or pumps milk which is frozen until the child can breastfeed.

Other conditions requiring surgery that are apparent shortly after birth include an imperforate anus, duodenal or jejunal obstructions, and malrotation or duplications in the small intestine.

Vomiting in infants

Both gastroesophageal reflux and pyloric stenosis in an infant can present as vomiting after feeding. Gastroesophageal reflux is a backward flow of gastric contents resulting in regurgitation or mild vomiting. It occurs more frequently in bottle-fed infants, which may be due to the differences in feeding position (breastfed infants are more erect during feeding) or pH.

Pyloric stenosis is the narrowing of the pylorus, the opening between the stomach and bowel. Infants with pyloric stenosis tend to have more violent projectile vomiting episodes after feeding causing dehydration and weight loss. They tend to overeat to compensate for these losses. The disorder is more prevalent in males, and no relationship to feeding method has yet been established. It can be treated by correction of dehydration and electrolyte imbalances followed by a pyloromyotomy.

GI tract abnormalities

The most frequent congenital abnormality of the colon is Hirschsprung's disease, also known as congenital aganglionic megacolon. It is found in some neonates who have a delayed passage of meconium. Initially the child is constipated and has a distended abdomen followed by vomiting because their peristaltic function is compromised by an absence of ganglion cells in muscles in the colon. A differential diagnosis must be done to distinguish Hirschsprung's disease from meconium ileus (usually a sign of cystic fibrosis), meconium plug syndrome, atresia of the ileus, or large bowel obstructions. A colostomy of the affected aganglionic region is performed, and breastfeeding, which is beneficial to these infants, can be started when the infant stabilizes.

A rare congenital abnormality is congenital chylothorax, which is the pleural effusion of the milky fluid called chyle (composed of lymph and fat) into the thoracic cavity. It can be life-threatening. Fluid must be drained from the infant's chest. Useful adjunctive therapies include parenteral nutrition, enteral feeding incorporating breast milk or formula, and mechanical ventilation.

- 67 -

Necrotizing enterocolitis

Necrotizing entercolitis (NEC) is death of intestinal tissue. This condition is generally found in premature infants or newborns that have been asphyxiated. It is often associated with exchange transfusions or infection with gram-negative bacteria including *Klebsiella*, *Escherichia coli*, and *Bacteroides*. Presentations include distension, vomiting, diarrhea, and blood in the stool. Current management protocols include stopping oral feedings, administration of antibiotics (oral and systemic), a septic workup, gastric decompression, and blood or plasma transfusions. Radiographs are done periodically to watch for perforations, which may indicate a colostomy or other surgery. Some researchers suggest that methods of stimulating bifidobacteria might be helpful because the infectious agents are suppressed. There is also some evidence, primarily in animal studies, that colostrum and breast milk may protect against NEC.

Gastrointestinal bleeding

If fresh blood is detected in the vomit or stool of a breastfed newborn, the first step is to identify the source of the blood. A qualitative assay in which blood is mixed with normal saline and approximately the same volume of 10% sodium hydroxide (NaOH) is performed. The color will change from pink to brown if the source is adult (presumably the mother through a cracked or bleeding nipple) but there is no color change if the source is fetal hemoglobin. If fetal Hb is indicated, then infant intestinal bleeding is occurring, and its cause must be determined. A cause cannot be found in about half the cases of infant GI bleeding. Hemorrhagic disorders account for about 20% of cases in newborns and other common causes are ingestion of maternal blood, anorectal fissures, and colitis. Colitis is a common source in older infants.

Breastfeeding before and after infant surgery

Infants requiring surgery can generally be breastfed up to 2 hours before and shortly after surgery. This is true even for cases of congenital heart disease. The main determining factor is the balance between the infant's ability to tolerate the anesthesia required (which would normally dictate up to 8 hours of pre-surgery withdrawal of feeding), the anxiety caused by separation from the mother, and expected feeding patterns. If the infant is older and needs to be rehospitalized past the neonatal period or if for some reason the mother cannot be with the child constantly, breast milk can be pumped and used later.

Sudden infant death syndrome

Sudden infant death syndrome (SIDS), the death of an apparently healthy infant usually during sleep, is responsible for a third of deaths during the first year of life. While the exact cause of SIDS is unknown, the negative associations identified are maternal smoking, infant sleeping in the prone position, infant sharing the bed, and not breastfeeding. Strategies to lower the incidence of sudden infant death syndrome include breastfeeding, use of pacifiers in infants who bottle feed, and other sleeping positions. Bed sharing increases the likelihood of infant death from being crushed or suffocated; even though some pediatricians feel bed sharing increases the bond between mother and child, the practice is not endorsed by the American Academy of Pediatrics.

Breastfeeding and tooth decay

Children who have been breastfed for unusually long periods, typically 2 to 3 years, often develop extensive tooth decay or dental caries. The association is even more pronounced if the frequency of nursing is great or the child breastfeeds at night. Breastfed infants have mutant streptococci in their oral cavity, the levels of which are elevated in children with extensive caries. They also have lactobacilli on their teeth. Dental caries are promoted by acid-forming bacteria and carbohydrate ingestion. They also have a familial component, which means children from families with a high incidence of tooth decay should receive fluoride treatments.

Failure-to-thrive

"Failure-to-thrive" is the term usually used to represent any infant who demonstrates some degree of growth failure. It is an imprecise term because there are various definitions that include parameters for weight, weight gain or loss, and height relative to percentile or percentage of median values. The generally accepted definition of failure-to-thrive is weight loss after day 10 of life, failure to reestablish birth weight by 3 weeks of age, or rate of weight gain less than the 10th percentile at age 1 month or more. Breastfed infants are more likely to be diagnosed with failure-to-thrive than those bottle-fed. The recommended median weight gain diminishes over the first year of life. During the first three months of life, babies should gain 26-31 g/day, and by ages 9 to 12 months, the expected gain is only 9 g/day. The difficulty with these averages is that growth is usually sporadic. Other experts consider growth as a continuum ranging from normal to varying degrees of malnutrition, with less than 60% of median weight considered severely malnourished rather than failure-to-thrive.

Difference from a slow gaining infant
A slow gaining infant is distinguished from one with failure-to-thrive by assessing various parameters. A slow gaining infant is alert and healthy with good muscle tone and skin turgor whereas one with failure-to-thrive is not healthy, appears lethargic, usually cries a lot, and has poor muscle tone and skin rigidity. Weight gain is slow but consistent in the slow gaining child, but the infant with failure-to-thrive has either irregular weight gain or weight loss. The feeding pattern is normal and frequent and the let-down reflex is functioning in slow weight gainers, but in infants with failure-to-thrive the feedings are limited (<8/day) and brief, and the let-down reflex is absent. This manifests as more wet diapers, pale and dilute urine, and usually frequent, seedy stools from the slow gaining infant. On the other hand, the baby with failure-to-thrive has few wet diapers, stronger urine, and sporadic, sparse stools. A nursing child can develop failure-to-thrive through maternal causes (poor production or let-down reflex) or because of their own diminished intake, low net intake because of intestinal issues or infection, or high energy requirements.

Underlying disorders
Infants being evaluated for failure-to-thrive should be examined for presence of underlying conditions that may cause poor sucking and swallowing. There are three types of disorders. The first type includes those in which there is an absent or diminished suck. The list of these is large, including neuromuscular abnormalities like kernicterus (bilirubin encephalopathy of the brain) and muscular dystrophy, infections affecting the central nervous system such as toxoplasmosis or bacterial meningitis; prematurity; hypoxia; hypothyroidism; and trisomy 21 or 13-15.

Additionally, the infant may be experiencing mechanical difficulties with suckling due to things like cleft lip, an enlarged tongue, or jaw or gum problems.

There are also a number of disorders that primarily affect the infant's ability to swallow, such as cleft palate, post-

- 69 -

intubation dysphasia, tumors or diverticula in the pharynx, or paralysis of the palate.

An intake problem unrelated to these identifiable underlying causes is termed either nonorganic failure-to-thrive or growth failure secondary to feeding skills disorder, probably related to some degree of oral sensorimotor impairment.

Small-for-gestational-age infants
An infant who is small-for-gestational-age (SGA) is one who despite full-term gestation has a low birth weight. SGA infants may develop failure-to-thrive. The first step in evaluation of the SGA child is to determine the reason intrauterine growth was small. Possibilities include maternal ailments or smoking, intrauterine infections, toxemia, and placental insufficiency. Intrauterine starvation makes the SGA child exhausted; thus they have difficulty suckling at first, which exacerbates eating issues. Any means to encourage successful breastfeeding should be employed, such as administration by tube or cup, lactation stimulating devices, and frequent feedings. The child has caloric requirements equivalent to a normal weight, full-term infant, which must be met to make up for intrauterine deprivation. In particular, breastfeeding can provide taurine and other essential amino acids and fats to promote brain growth.

Metabolic insufficiencies and situations with high energy requirements
The law requires metabolic screening of newborns, which can identify disorders of metabolism that may contribute to failure-to-thrive. Some of the metabolic disorders that can cause failure-to-thrive are hypothyroidism, phenylketonuria (PKU), hyperbilirubinemia, and galactosemia. High levels of total serum bilirubin are usually accompanied by jaundice (or more serious brain accumulation) and can be critical in newborns. Underfeeding and starvation can lead to breastfeeding jaundice in infants above 3 days of age. Galactosemia is an inherited disorder in which galactose-1-phosphate uridyltransferase activity is diminished and galactose cannot be metabolized resulting in weight loss, jaundice, and other problems. The child must not consume lactose, thus necessitating weaning. Infants with central nervous system disorders or congestive heart disease, those who were born small-for-gestational-age, or those who may be exposed to maternal stimulants through breast milk all tend to have high energy requirements.

Low net intake
Low net intake is related to loss through vomiting and diarrhea, gastrointestinal malabsorption, or infections. Diarrhea and vomiting are rare in breastfed infants, but they can be associated with underlying pyloric stenosis, metabolic disorders, food allergies, or intake of excessive fruit juice. An infant with low growth can be experiencing an acute infection of the gastrointestinal tract, evidenced by looking at the stools, or the urinary tract, which can be identified using urinalysis and white blood cell and differential counts. Infants who were infected in utero may be born small-for-gestational age, which, as discussed elsewhere, predisposes them to failure-to-thrive. In addition, some chronic viral infections, such as hepatitis, AIDS, or CMV can manifest as failure-to-thrive.

Prolonged exclusive breastfeeding
Nonorganic failure-to-thrive (NOFTT), in which there is no apparent organic cause for infant growth failure, can often be attributed to prolonged, exclusive breastfeeding past age 6 months. Children with normal weight gain during the first year of life and suddenly have poor weight increases or losses may be experiencing NOFTT. Breast milk alone

- 70 -

does not provide the nutrition needed for growth after this age. Solids add needed protein and minerals, like iron and zinc. Many experts feel that psychological factors, such as retention of maternal control over feeding, contribute to this type of NOFTT; it is sometimes called reactive attachment disorder. A variation is vulnerable child syndrome in which similar poor growth occurs in older infants who breastfeed often and take in a minimum of other foods.

Maternal causes

Maternal causes of infant failure-to-thrive are related to either poor production of milk or an inadequate let-down reflex. Poor or less nutritious milk production can be due to anatomic, hormonal, pharmacologic, nutritional, or stress-producing factors. There are rare instances of lactation failure due to inadequate glandular development in the breast or a retained placenta. Mothers who are malnourished or restrict their diets below suggested lactation energy or protein levels may not provide enough nourishment for the infant through breastfeeding. The pattern of breastfeeding can be important since mothers who feed with only one breast eventually produce milk that is higher in fat content (thus promoting growth) than milk from two-breast feeding. The most frequent cause of poor milk production is maternal fatigue, which is a stressor along with maternal illness. An inadequate let-down reflex (suppression of oxytocin release) can be caused by smoking, medications such as L-dopa, or psychological factors; an oxytocin nasal spray may be helpful to stimulating the let-down reflex.

Dehydration and electrolyte complications

Severe dehydration accompanied by hypernatremia is an emergency situation. It can occur when effective breastfeeding has not been established. Dehydration can diagnosed by observation of poor skin turgor and tone; and elevated concentrations of blood urea nitrogen (BUN), creatinine, hematocrit, and urinary specific gravity. Electrolyte levels should also be examined. About half of presenting dehydrated infants also have hypernatremia, abnormally high serum sodium concentrations, as a result of hypernatremic mother's milk. Hypernatremic dehydration responds to increased lactation (which eventually produces milk with lower sodium concentrations) and sometimes intravenous fluids in efforts to normalize the infant's sodium levels. Severe dehydration has also been associated with chloride deficiency syndrome in the infant.

Pharmacology and Toxicology

Drugs in breast milk

Ability of drugs to pass into breast milk

Women take various drugs during pregnancy, labor, and postpartum. The ability of these drugs to pass into human breast milk and potentially to the infant through breastfeeding depends on a variety of factors. The route of delivery (oral, intravenous, intramuscular, subcutaneous, or transdermal) influences the ability of the drug to get into the milk. Properties of the drug such as its absorption rate, molecular weight, half-life, the dissociation constant, volume distribution in the body, the degree to which the drug is ionized, protein binding properties, solubility of the drug in water versus lipids, and the pH of the drug and substrate all affect the drug's availability. In general, less drug reaches the mammary alveolar cells and breast milk than is found in the plasma; in other words the milk/plasma (M/P) ratio is less than 1 for most drugs.

Protein binding and ionization properties of drugs

Drugs are absorbed into the bloodstream in both unbound (free drug) and protein-bound forms and then distributed to various tissues. They can be metabolized in the liver, interact in some way with the brain, stored in bone and fat tissues, or excreted via the kidneys or breast milk. Only free molecules can pass from plasma to milk via simple or carrier-assisted diffusion or active transport to endothelial pores. Thus the concentration of the drug is usually lower in milk than in plasma. The ionization properties of the drug also affect its milk levels since excreted drugs are generally in non-ionized form. Since the pH of plasma (7.4) is higher than that of milk (6.8-7.3), drugs or compounds that are weakly acidic are more ionized and protein-bound in plasma and do not pass as easily into milk as do mildly alkaline drugs or compounds. The degree of ionization is also related to the dissociation constant (pK_a), with a higher pK_a increasing the milk/plasma (M/P) ratio.

Solubility and molecular weight properties of drugs

Drugs are primarily water or lipid soluble. In order to be present in breast milk, the drug must pervade the membrane of the alveolar epithelial cells, which is made up of various forms of lipids. The mammary alveolar epithelium is optimally permeable during colostrum production. Drugs that are highly soluble in lipids, such as those in non-ionized form pass easily into the breast milk. Non-ionized drugs can have a milk/plasma ratio of about 1.0 and are eliminated at a rate equal to that found in plasma. Drugs that are less soluble in lipids do not pass as much into the milk, but they do not clear as quickly either. Those that are highly protein-bound in the mother's serum do not significantly cross the barrier into breast milk. Water-soluble drugs and ions cannot penetrate the alveolar epithelium's lipid barrier, and only small molecular weight versions (up to MW 200) can diffuse through pores in the basement membrane or spaces between cells.

Mechanisms of transport and concentrations

Drug molecules can pass from plasma into breast milk through simple passive diffusion to equalize the concentration gradient. Diffusion across the cell membrane can also be facilitated by proteins or enzymes that aid the transfer; this method aids transport of larger molecular weight water-soluble compounds. Another mechanism is the active transport of substances that are already in high concentrations in milk. Active transport is achieved through use of membrane pumps, pinocytosis, or reverse pinocytosis. Pinocytosis is the intake of fluid through attachment to cell membrane receptors and inward folding and pinching off of the fluid and membrane portion into the cell. In reverse pinocytosis, the plasma membrane fuses with membrane-bound granules, folds outward, and pinches off into the alveolar lumen.

Drugs in plasma and other compartments

Pharmacokinetics of drug distribution

Pharmacokinetics refers to the body's reaction to and distribution following drug intake. The concentrations of a drug found in plasma and other compartments are influenced by the route of administration and the patterns of absorption, metabolism, distribution, and elimination. The volume of distribution (V_d) is the pattern of drug distribution. If the body were a single uniform compartment, then simple first-order kinetics could be used to define the volume of distribution as the total amount of drug in the body divided by its concentration in plasma. In this simplified version, the expected drug concentration in breast milk would be the dose given divided by the V_d. In reality, the calculation is much more complex, as drugs are assimilated or stored in other tissues besides the breast, and breast milk levels are influenced by factors such as the drug's dissociation constant, pH, protein-binding capacity, solubility, and the relative rates of excretion through lactation versus back diffusion into plasma.

Administration route

If a drug is delivered through intravenous bolus, its plasma levels quickly peak and then fall off. If the route of administration is intramuscularly (or subcutaneously), the drug is absorbed and clears more slowly. Single oral dosing has a predictable plasma concentration curve, but multiple dosing is less straightforward and other factors such as the relationship to meals can affect plasma levels. Drugs are often given using a transdermal drug delivery system (TDDS), which uses a reservoir (often a patch) in the epidermis to distribute the drug through the skin. TDDS theoretically offers a constant rate of delivery and a consistent plasma drug level while the patch is worn. Some of the most common TDDS systems are for delivery of scopolamine (for motion sickness or sedation), nicotine (for smoking withdrawal), clonidine (for hypertension), and fentanyl (a narcotic given for pain). Certain nicotine and clonidine patches can deliver drug amounts to the infant that are toxic.

Response of infant to drugs

The effects of maternal drugs on the infant during nursing are primarily influenced by two factors. The first is the rate of absorption from the gastrointestinal tract into the child's bloodstream, which is dependent on several aspects such as milk volume, oral bioavailability of the drug, and breakdown in the GI tract. The second is the infant's facility to detoxify and excrete the drug. This means the infant's ability to bind the drug to proteins in the liver or some alternative pathway and then excrete the conjugate via urine or stool. Drugs that do not conjugate can build up in the infant's system and have untoward effects. The gestational age at birth can influence the infant's ability to detoxify and excrete the drug. This is because less mature infants have high water content and lower amounts of protein available for binding to the drug. Acidosis and hypoxia during premature delivery can also displace protein (albumin) binding

- 73 -

creating more free drug in the infant's circulation. Less mature infants are not as capable of metabolizing drugs in the liver and clearing them through the kidneys.

Importance of milk volume and fat content

Older infants generally consume more breast milk than younger ones depending on the nutritional contribution from other food sources. If the total consumed breast milk approaches a liter of milk daily, significant amounts of drugs can be passed to the infant via breast milk. Fat content of milk fluctuates, which can influence the effects of lipid-soluble drugs in the milk. Generally, milk at the beginning of the feeding (foremilk) is lower in fat content than later milk (hindmilk). Fat content is also cyclical, with peak levels found at midday. The permeability and concentrations of lipid-soluble drugs are related to fat content. Drugs that are not particularly fat-soluble are present in the aqueous and protein portions of the milk, meaning they are more likely to be present in foremilk or during periods of lower fat content.

Assessing possible effects of drugs

One of the most important issues to discuss when administering drugs to a nursing mother is whether the drug is safe for direct administration to the infant. This can be impacted by factors such as the expected dosage actually reaching the child, the amount of enzyme induction that has taken place in utero, and the length of time the drug is to be taken by the mother. To estimate dose delivered to the infant, use the following calculation.

Dose to infant in 24 hours = concentration in milk x infant weight (kg) x volume of milk ingested/kg in 24 hours.
The oral availability of the drug, in other words, the percentage of drug absorbed

in the infant's gut, should also be considered; thus, drugs or administration routes that result in low oral bioavailability are safer. Other assessment considerations are the possibility of food-drug interactions and the risk of development of drug sensitivities or resistance. If there is little information about the drug's safety during pregnancy and/or lactation, prudence in use should be observed. The breastfed child should be watched carefully if the mother is taking drugs. Every attempt to minimize excretion into or accumulation in breast milk should be taken. Therefore, it is advisable to take drug therapies after breastfeeding and avoid long-lasting or extended release preparations.

Classification systems for drugs used during lactation

The National Swedish Board of Health and other organizations group drugs taken during lactation into four categories based on whether the active ingredients enter the milk and the amounts transferred. Group I includes those agents that do not pass active drug to the milk. Group II drugs enter the milk but in small quantities that do not pose a risk to the child. Group III includes agents that are present in milk in greater and potentially harmful amounts. Group IV (about half) agents have unknown activity or effect on breast milk. The American Academy of Pediatrics takes a different approach by listing 7 drug categories in which the relationship of approximately 300 drugs to breastfeeding is defined. The classifications are: (1) cytotoxic drugs, (2) drugs of abuse, (3) radioactive compounds, (4) drugs of concern with unknown effects on infants, (5) medications anecdotally implicated as affecting nursing infants, (6) drugs appropriate to breastfeeding, and (7) food and environmental agents.

Maternal use of drugs and effects on infants

Analgesics

An analgesic is any pain-relieving medication that does not cause loss of consciousness. Analgesics can pass into breast milk. The milder types that are usually available over the counter (such as aspirin, ibuprofen and acetaminophen) or often prescribed (such as codeine) can be used in moderation by the mother without adversely affecting the child. Mothers usually take single doses of aspirin for pain. Even with more frequent doses, the metabolite salicylate, not acetylsalicylic acid, which can cause platelet aggregation problems, is found in the newborn. The infant can metabolize acetaminophen well, and ibuprofen has such a short half-life that little reaches the infant via breast milk. The narcotic fentanyl citrate is cleared quickly, and codeine is only present in milk in low levels. Short-acting analgesics like nalbuphine or butorphanol, which may be used during labor, have been associated with an enhanced ability of the infant to establish breastfeeding. Epidural anesthesia has been associated with postpartum complications.

Antibiotics

Antibiotic use is often contraindicated in nursing mothers. In many cases, the mother should not take a drug until the child is old enough to take it directly without impunity. Some classes of antibiotics are relatively harmless, such as aminoglycosides, which are not readily absorbed in the infant's GI tract, and cephalosporins, which have poor oral absorption. Some drugs that can pose problems are penicillin (which may cause sensitivity), sulfa drugs (which can impede binding of bilirubin to protein), tetracycline (which can cause discoloration of teeth and problems with bone growth), erythromycin (which can interfere with clearance of other drugs), and the anti-protozoal medication metronidazole (Flagyl, used for vaginal infections).

Gastrointestinal medications

The H_2-receptor antagonist cimetidine (Tagamet) passes readily into breast milk, probably through some sort of active transport mechanism. The drug, which is indicated for gastric acidity, gastroesophageal reflux, or gastric ulcers, should be used cautiously even though it has been designated as compatible with breastfeeding. Other medications used for gastric acidity, such as famotidine and omeprazole, are fairly safe because they have low milk levels and low oral bioavailability. Sulfasalazine, which is used to treat ulcerative colitis and Crohn's disease, is also harmless because its metabolites are absorbed from the colon and broken down in the liver or excreted in the urine.

Anticoagulants

Anticoagulants are agents administered to reduce the possibility of blood clotting. The two major anticoagulants are heparin and warfarin. Structurally, heparins are glycosaminoglycans, chains composed of D-glucosamine and uronic acid, which can be of varying lengths. The low-molecular-weight (LMW) forms of heparin are generally given. Because of their large size (a molecular weight of at least 2000), LMW heparins cannot pass into breast milk or cross the placenta. Therefore, they can be safely given to the mother without affecting the child. Warfarin, a coumarin derivative, has not been shown to pass into breast milk, and some experts consider its use preferable in the lactating mother.

Anticholinergic drugs

Anticholinergic drugs block the neurotransmitter acetylcholine and, therefore, nerve impulses. Some of the most commonly administered anticholinergic drugs, atropine and scopolamine, both pass into breast milk. Atropine, utilized as a muscle relaxant, can suppress milk production and cause a rapid heart rate, thermal changes, constipation, or urinary retention in the child. Scopolamine is usually administered via a TDDS dermal patch for motion sickness; its major side effect is that it tends to dry the mother's mucous membranes. Both atropine and scopolamine are nevertheless rated by the American Academy of Pediatrics as category 6, generally acceptable in conjunction with breastfeeding. The anticholinergic drug class also includes synthetic quaternary ammonium derivatives such as mepenzolate methylbromide.

Antithyroid drugs
Antithyroid drugs are hormone antagonists that block thyroid activity. Three of the more common drugs used for hyperthyroidism or overactive thyroid (thiouracil, methimazole, and carbimazole) present potential risks to the breastfeeding child. These include possible infant thyroid suppression and goiter (enlarged thyroid). The maternal milk to plasma ratio (M/P) is much greater than 1 for thiouracil, indicating active transport mechanisms and probability of transmission to the child. Thus, maternal use during lactation should be cautioned. Studies have also shown significant amounts of methimazole and carbimazole in the mother's milk. Some experts believe that another antithyroid drug, propylthiouracil (PTU), is the drug of choice because it does not appear to pass as readily into the breast milk. The newborn's thyroid function should be monitored if these drugs are taken by the mother. Iodide has a high M/P ratio and should be avoided because it can cause goiter or sensitivity to other drug classes.

Methylxanthines
Methylxanthines are methylated xanthine derivatives. The most commonly consumed methylxanthine is caffeine. Excessive maternal caffeine ingestion can cause hyperactivity in the nursing infant. Some caffeine does pass into and can accumulate in breast milk. Another methylxanthine, theobromine is found in chocolate and cocoa-containing products. Several other methylxanthines are used by asthmatics as bronchodilators. These include theophylline and dyphylline, both of which are found in breast milk and can be passed into the child's circulation. Other types of asthma treatments, particularly inhalants, may be indicated for the mother. Examples include inhaled albuterol (a beta-2-adrenergic agonist) and inhaled or nasal spray forms of the corticosteroid fluticasone.

Drugs of abuse and alcohol

Drugs of abuse, specifically cocaine, heroin, marijuana, amphetamine, and phencyclidine hydrochloride, are rated Category 2 by the AAP and should not be taken during breastfeeding. Alcohol (rated as AAP Category 6) should be consumed in moderation and relative to feeding. Various studies indicate that small amounts, less than 1 g alcohol/kg weight, of alcohol are safe. Higher levels of alcohol can depress the let-down reflex or prevent milk-ejection by blocking oxytocin release. Alcohol does pass into the breast milk and can cause a distinctive odor to the milk. Infants tend to suck less efficiently and may have sleeping problems if they ingest alcohol-containing breast milk. Alcohol consumption during pregnancy may increase the risk of having a low birth weight child.

Herbs and herbal teas

At present, herbal medicine is the utilization of unprocessed natural plant constituents to treat ailments. Many herbs are believed to be beneficial, but few claims regarding such are substantiated. Herbal concoctions are also classified as dietary supplements, which are not regulated by the Food and Drug Administration. The only types of herbal teas that are considered safe for lactating mothers are those containing strictly chicory, orange spice, peppermint, raspberry, red blush, and/or rose hips. Preparations of ginger or peppermint, which have been touted for reduction of nausea and vomiting during pregnancy, may not be safe at high doses.

Mother's milk tea
Mother's milk tea is a preparation that has been touted as a promoter of lactation. It does not contain caffeine but still produces euphoria and other side effects. While some of the ingredients are galactagogues, such as blessed thistle leaf and fenugreek seed, many have potentially toxic effects. These include fennel seed, a weak diuretic that can affect the central nervous system; chamomile flower, which can act as an antispasmodic but can also cause vomiting and vertigo; and comfrey leaf (addressed elsewhere), which can cause venoocclusive disease and hepatotoxicity. Relatively safe ingredients include coriander seed, which increases saliva and gastric juice flow; lemongrass for flavoring; borage leaves, which act as diuretics and euphorics; and star anise (a mild stimulant and expectorant). Even the galactagogues have potential side effects, mainly vomiting (blessed thistle leaf) and hypoglycemia or induction of labor (fenugreek seed).

Potential side effects of herbal teas
Herbal teas that contain ephedra are contraindicated because the herb can cause hypertension, rapid heartbeat, and even death. Tea tree oil, which is applied topically to treat fungal infections, can cause contact dermatitis and muscle weakness and should never be ingested.

The sedative comfrey is discussed elsewhere as a promoter of venoocclusive disease and hepatic failure; pennyroyal can also cause hepatic failure, renal failure, and spontaneous abortion. Teas containing aconite can precipitate cardiac irregularities, nausea, and neuromuscular weakness leading to seizures or coma. Aloe vera, generally applied topically as a gel for a variety of reasons, can cause diarrhea, gastric cramping, and contact dermatitis. Allergic responses have been documented to chamomile and feverfew in herbal teas. Goldenseal, generally used for diarrhea or as an antiseptic, can influence blood pressure, induce GI problems, and increase the amount of free bilirubin by displacement; it is should not be used in infants. No side effects have been reported for the immunostimulant echinacea.

Toxicities in herbal teas
Comfrey leaf, or *Symphytum officinate*, which is typically included in mother's milk tea and also found in other forms, is potentially very dangerous to a fetus or breastfeeding infant. The leaves can cause fetal death due to venoocclusive disease; they contain high levels of pyrrolizidine alkaloids, which can cause liver toxicity; and they also have carcinogenic potential. Another herb that contains the same alkaloids and therefore has similar possible effects is thread-leafed groundsel, or *Senecio longilobus.* The aromatic oil safrole, which is found in sassafras and herbal teas, is potentially carcinogenic, toxic to the central nervous system, and interactive with other drugs; it is prohibited by the FDA in regulated preparations. There have been cases where natural coumarin, such as those found in sweet clover, have caused hemorrhaging. Lactating mothers should not consume large amounts of licorice because it has been found to cause hypertension, sodium retention, and depressed potassium levels.

Herbal medicines discontinued before surgery

There are 8 herbal medicines contraindicated for use before surgery. Ginseng and garlic should be withdrawn at least a week before the surgery. Ginseng lowers blood glucose levels and inhibits platelet aggregation predisposing the individual to hypoglycemia and the risk of bleeding; it is contraindicated during lactation as well. Garlic impedes platelet aggregation and increases fibrinolysis, again raising the possibility of bleeding. St. John's wort (hypericum) is an antidepressant that inhibits neurotransmitter uptake. It should not be taken for at least 5 days prior to surgery because it induces cytochrome P450 enzymes and interacts with a number of drug types; it can also suppress lactation. Gingko, which inhibits platelet-activating factor, is another herb that should be discontinued several days before surgery due to its potential for inducing bleeding. Herbals that should be stopped 24 hours prior to surgery are ephedra (which increases heart rate and blood pressure and could cause numerous cardiovascular problems), the sedatives kava and valerian, and echinacea (an activator of cell-mediated immunity).

Psychoactive substances in herbal preparations

Herbal preparations have gained popularity in recent years. Many of the herbs included have psychoactive properties. Some are stimulants or mild hallucinogens; examples include kava kava, mandrake, passion flower, juniper, and others. Others are sedatives or tranquilizers, such as scotch broom, hops, and valerian. Several can cause allergic reactions, including Burdock root (which can prompt anaphylactic shock due to its atropine-like effects) and chamomile (which can cause contact dermatitis). Comfrey leaves and groundsel can precipitate venoocclusive disease and hepatic failure. Others, like woodruff, can cause hemorrhaging. The list of potentially harmful herbs is long.

Galactagogues

Galactagogues are substances that can induce lactation. Controlled clinical trials of drugs and herbal preparations used as galactagogues have not been done but anecdotal information exists. The most extensively studied lactation promoting drug is the domperidone (often used for nausea or indigestion). It can have adverse effects such as arrhythmias, neurological effects, dry mouth, and abdominal cramps. Metoclopramide is an antiemetic drug, which is used to induce lactation through promotion of prolactin release; it should only be used with caution for a limited amount of time. It is also given to infants to treat reflux but is controversial because it can accumulate in the infant's system.

Many herbs are anecdotally considered galactagogues. Fenugreek is among the safer choices when used in moderation. Some herbs have been noted to promote other effects that enhance but do not actually promote lactation, such as grapefruit seed extract, which has anti-infectious properties and may be useful topically for sore nipples. Claims for other herbs are largely unsubstantiated, or the herb may have harmful consequences.

Lactation suppressants

Compounds that suppress lactation are generally those that have a drying effect. Decongestants, particularly pseudoephedrine, have been found to suppress lactation. The mechanism is not entirely clear as significant amounts of pseudoephedrine have not been demonstrated in breast milk and the drug does not appear to affect prolactin levels. The family of sage plants, which are used both as flavorings and medicinally, have been shown to suppress lactation and reduce sweating. The herb can be used to decrease milk supply when appropriate, such as in attempts to speed up the weaning process or treat breast engorgement.

Use of drugs during pregnancy and lactation

Cardiovascular drugs
Digitalis, a cardiotonic medication used for congestive heart failure and other cardiac problems, is passed into milk; nursing mothers should avoid nursing during the period of peak concentrations (1 ½-3 hours after administration of the drug). A number of anti-hypertensive drugs have high milk to plasma ratios and should be used cautiously while breastfeeding. The safest anti-hypertensive choice is metoprolol, which has a milk to plasma ratio of less than 1. The drug reserpine, also used to treat high blood pressure, should not be used during pregnancy or breastfeeding. Propranolol, a beta-adrenergic blocker, can be transmitted to breast milk as well; if used by the mother, the infant should be checked for signs of hypoglycemia and plasma levels of the drug.

Diuretics
Diuretics are drugs that increase the excretion of urine. They are also used to relieve hypertension. Generally nursing mothers can take diuretics as they are weak acids and negligibly transferred to breast milk. They also tend to have short half-lives in the mother so careful timing relative to breastfeeding can minimize passage of the drug to the infant. The most concerning problem presented by diuretics, in particular chlorothiazide and furosemide, is their ability to generate free bilirubin through displacement of bilirubin-albumin complexes. Some diuretics, such as the agent chlorthalidone, can suppress milk production.

Drugs that affect the central nervous system
Most drugs that affect the central nervous system (CNS) have high milk to plasma (M/P) ratios. These include phenobarbital, primidone, diphenylhydantoin, and carbamazepine. They also have relatively long half-lives in infants. If they are taken by the mother, infant plasma levels should be checked after a week or two of breastfeeding to monitor accretion.

There are reports that anti-convulsant drug use can hamper lactation and cause prolonged infant suckling difficulty. Another CNS drug, valproic acid, is not found in significant amounts in breast milk but it does have a long infant half-life.

The anti-epileptic drug phenytoin has been associated with infant vomiting, tremors, rashes, and other side effects, but it usually is not problematic as the amounts of drug transmitted to the child are far below therapeutic levels.

Psychotherapeutic agents
Psychotherapeutic agents used to treat depression and other neurological issues can be problematic due to the long-term therapeutic regimens and possible transfer to breast milk. Risk-benefit scenarios should be carefully considered before initiating treatment during pregnancy or lactation.

The most popular psychotherapeutic agents are selective serotonin reuptake inhibitors (SSRIs); SSRIs include fluoxetine (Prozac), paroxetine (Paxil), sertraline (Zoloft,) and others. Fluoxetine is one of the least dangerous in terms of transmission to breast milk and the infant.

Tricyclic antidepressants, such as imipramine and clomipramine, can pass into breast milk because they are lipid-

- 79 -

soluble; the AAP considers their concerning (Category 4).

Lithium should not be taken during pregnancy.

Diazepam (Valium) and chlordiazepoxide (Librium) have been associated with adverse effects in breastfeeding infants. One of the safer choices of psychotropic agents is chlorpromazine.

Methadone

People with heroin and other opiate addictions are commonly placed on a maintenance scheme of daily methadone, a synthetic narcotic drug. Methadone use during pregnancy at typical levels of 100-150 mg/day is problematic for the neonate, who is likely to experience withdrawal symptoms. The newborn may need to remain hospitalized for up to 2 weeks during their withdrawal. If the pregnant woman uses lower levels of methadone, for example 25 mg/day, infant withdrawal can be minimized. Maternal methadone maintenance during breastfeeding is considered Category 6, usually compatible with breastfeeding. Methadone is found in the breast milk, peaking at 4-5 hours after administration, suggesting that milk produced during that time period should be discarded. The actual concentration reaching the child is low relative to maternal intake, no untoward effects in infants have been demonstrated during breastfeeding or weaning, and weaning does not appear to result in infant withdrawal symptoms.

Environmental contaminants

Pesticides and pollutants

A number of organic pesticides and pollutants and their metabolites can be found in breast milk. These include chlorinated hydrocarbons like dichlorodiphenyltrichloroethane (DDT), polychlorinated and polybrominated biphenyls (PCBs and PBBs respectively),

heterocyclic hydrocarbons of the dioxin class (notably Agent Orange), flammable solvents called furans, and polybrominated diphenylethers (PBDEs, used as flame retardants). These chemicals pass easily into breast milk because they have an affinity for lipids, are found in non-ionized form at physiological pH, and have relatively low molecular weights. Exposure to these compounds depends in large part on the geographical region in which one lives. Heavy maternal exposure can be problematic for the infant; for example PBDE contact during pregnancy has been associated with cognitive and behavioral problems in the child. Most experts believe that breastfeeding by women with demonstrated pesticide or pollutant contact is usually more beneficial than the risk of infant exposure.

Heavy metals

Lead, mercury, arsenic, cadmium, and other heavy metals have been found in human breast milk. Local water supplies contain certain heavy metals, which can show up in formulas mixed with the water as well as in the lactating mother or nursing child. The heavy metals of greatest concern are lead and mercury. Lead poisoning can adversely affect a child's IQ. Peak concentrations of lead in the nursing mother occur 6-8 months after delivery due to skeletal reabsorption. Blood lead levels less than 10 ug/dL are safe (Class I), but increasing levels warrant prevention activities, more frequent community screening, and medical evaluations. A level of 45-69 ug/dL (Class IV) necessitates medical intervention, including chelation therapy and environmental intercession. A blood lead level greater than 69 ug/DL indicates a medical emergency. Mercury, which is primary found in fish, can be found in inorganic or relatively inaccessible organic forms attached to red blood cells (methylmercury); studies evaluating infant development suggest breastfeeding is advantageous over formula in the latter case.

Well water and workplace chemicals
Well water, which may be consumed by mothers in rural areas, contains a number of minerals. The mineral of most concern is nitrate, which is related to nitric acid and is often found in various fertilizers. Nitrate levels of more than 100 mg/L can cause methemoglobinemia, the presence of an altered form of hemoglobin that cannot bind oxygen, in infants predisposing them to hypoxia and death. High nitrate levels are a greater concern for formula-fed infants (due to mixing formula with water) than breastfed children.

Mothers who return to workplaces in which they may be exposed to volatile chemicals can place their child at risk for exposure. Protective gear should be worn to minimize exposure; these compounds are organic and have an affinity for lipids. The exact relationship between individual chemicals and infant exposure through breast milk is governed by both the pharmacokinetics of the compound and the blood/air partition coefficient, which determines the effects to the body. The EPA considers bromo chloromethane, perchloroethylene, and 1,4 –dioxane among the riskiest chemicals.

Radioactive materials
A nursing mother may be exposed to radioactive materials through diagnostic tests or therapeutic use of these agents. In all cases, there is some period after exposure in which the mother should discard milk and not breastfeed. The period of withdrawal depends on the amount of exposure, the half-life of the radioisotope used, and the rate of clearance from the milk. Diagnostic tests using radioactive materials typically require discontinuation of breastfeeding for 1-7 days. Therapeutic use can warrant breastfeeding cessation for up to 3 months. Radioisotopes of iodine (either ^{125}I or ^{131}I) have shown as much as a 5% transfer rate to breast milk. Other commonly utilized radioisotopes include ^{67}Ga (gallium) and ^{99m}Tc (technetium). Diagnostic procedures not requiring use of radioisotopes, such as ultrasound, computed tomography, or magnetic resonance imaging, are preferred.

Medications used during labor or delivery

Sedatives used during labor may transiently affect the suckling ability of a newborn for several days. These drugs include secobarbital and meperidine. Some studies also suggest that prolonged or repeated administration of epidural anesthesia during delivery may disturb infant feeding ability. Metabolites of anesthetics like fentanyl and bupivacaine have been found in neonatal urine. If meperidine is used in conjunction with an anesthetic, neurobehavioral parameters like alertness and suckling are depressed in the newborn. Chloroprocaine is a better choice for epidural anesthetic than bupivacaine because it is more rapidly broken down. Bupivacaine use has been associated with depressed alertness for a month following delivery.

Psychology, Sociology and Anthropology

Mother-infant interaction after delivery

If a healthy newborn is delivered to an unmedicated mother and immediately put on the mother's stomach prior to cutting the cord, quick bonding is initiated by the child within about 45 min. The alert infant will inch toward the mother's breast, find the nipple, latch on, and suckle without any assistance. If the mother has been medicated during labor, the newborn has more difficulty finding the breast and suckling. If the neonate is temporarily taken away from the mother after delivery, he/she is much more likely to cry until reunifications with the mother. Mothers allowed early contact with their newborn tend to nurse much longer and in a more attached fashion, and their infants are heavier and less prone to infection.

Cultural influences on body contact and nursing

Body contact and the length of nursing between mother and child are highly influenced by cultural traditions and perceptions. Cultural practices, climate, attitudes toward breast exposure, and perceptions about infant development versus time of weaning all play roles in the amount of contact between the pair and the time of weaning. Cultural traditions can dictate the way in which a child is carried; for example, soft carriers such as pouches or slings provide more opportunities for contact than cradleboards or crib use. Certain cultures encourage bed sharing with the parent, whereas others are more concerned with issues that demand less contact, such as sudden infant death syndrome. Mothers from high contact cultures tend to carry their children continuously during the first few months, wear minimal clothing, and allow bed sharing. Mothers from low contact cultures tend to separate the infant at birth, swaddle or heavily cloth the infant, use a crib or cradleboard, and sleep separately from the child.

Safe sleeping environment

The Academy of Breastfeeding Medicine has established some guidelines to ensure a safe sleeping environment for the bed sharing infant. Some salient features of the recommendations include using firm and flat surfaces for the sleeping, clothing or draping the infant in a sleeper or thin blanket, and having the infant lie on their back. They also suggest pillows and other possible dangers, such as stuffed animals or comforters be removed from the immediate environment, and there should be no spaces that allow infant falls or suffocation. An infant should never be placed alone on an adult bed.

Unrestricted and token breastfeeding

Unrestricted breastfeeding refers to frequent, on-demand breastfeeding by the mother without regard to timing. Bottle-feeding is not offered and solid introduction is delayed until after age 6 months. Token breastfeeding is the practice of feeding according to predetermined frequency and length. Generally children who are token breastfed wean earlier (usually by month 3) and bottle-feeding or occasional solid introduction may occur. Token breastfeeding may be accompanied by poor establishment of the let-down reflex, engorgement, and behavioral issues with the child. These definitions encompass the psychological differences related to breastfeeding style, while newer classifications call them exclusive versus partial breastfeeding. Studies have demonstrated personality differences between mothers receptive to unrestricted nursing, versus those who token breastfeed and bottle feed. The latter tend be conflicted as to the role of nursing or see the breast as more of a sexual organ.

Differences between breastfeeding and bottle-feeding

There are varied measureable differences between breastfeeding and bottle-feeding women. The breast of a lactating woman is warmer than one who is not. A number of parameters that indicate stress, including plasma levels of adrencorticotropic hormone, cortisol and epinephrine as well as a perceived level of lower stress, are depressed in lactating versus non-lactating women. After breastfeeding, lactating mothers present with elevated mood (assessed by the Positive and Negative Affect Scale), which is probably a result of oxytocin production during let-down. Objective parameters need to be considered within the larger context of cultural influences and personal choice.

Human imprinting and nipple substitutes

Human imprinting refers to a rapid learning process that occurs early in life and establishes later behavioral patterns. In the context of breastfeeding, the term is concerned with the seeking out of a particular set of stimuli, in this case, the shape of the nipple. If an infant suckles on a rubber bottle nipple, pacifier, part of their hand/thumb, or other object, the child can confuse the nipple-like source with their mother's breast. Use of the thumb, a pacifier or an empty bottle is non-nutritive sucking whereas suckling the breast or a filled nursing bottle is nutritive (distinctions discussed elsewhere).

Relationship between breastfeeding style and let-down reflex

A mother who practices unrestricted breastfeeding immediately triggers the let-down reflex and has a swollen breast upon hearing her child cry. This occurs because these children do not cry much otherwise, the mother is generally less stressed, and both oxytocin release and maternal behaviors are more spontaneous. The mother who practices token breastfeeding feeds on schedule and without correlation to her milk supply. Token breastfed children tend to be more agitated. The mother is therefore likely to experience more stress and less likely to release oxytocin to trigger the let-down reflex. Bottle-fed infants and mothers have been shown to experience more anxiety, depression, and fatigue than either breastfeeding group. Evidence suggests that breastfeeding can relax and provide emotional gratification to the mother.

Psychological impact of breastfeeding

<u>On infant</u>
Breastfeeding provides time for more social interaction and a greater feeling of control experienced by the infant than bottle-feeding. Breastfed newborns are more attentive and active. Children who were breastfed have long-term developmental advantages as well, such as the tendency to walk earlier and score higher on achievement tests. Those children who are nursed longer show better performance to a point; if exclusive breastfeeding is continued past one year, the advantages are reversed. The relationship between breastfeeding, personality, and ability to adjust as an infant and in later life is complex and hard to define. Various studies have shown a reverse correlation between duration of breastfeeding and disorderly conduct in school, higher degrees of anxiety in women who were bottle-fed as infants,

and a high level of stress related to abrupt weaning. Mothers who are forced to wean abruptly may experience postpartum depression at that time.

On family members
Various studies support the notion that the father should be an active participant in the birthing process as well as while the mother is breastfeeding. Early involvement of the father translates to greater paternal participation in the future. Some see the father's role as that of a coach while others envision him more as a source of encouragement and physical assistance. Nonnutritive hugging and comforting of the child are important parts of the father's role. Some men do have difficulty defining their function while their wife is nursing because they feel they cannot participate as actively or they have conflicts regarding their partner's breast in both a sexual and familial context. The father's perceptions about the nursing process and his role have been demonstrated to affect the success and length of breastfeeding. Less is known about the impact of the mother's breastfeeding on other siblings. The woman's attitudes toward privacy requirements and the like can surely affect the other children's viewpoints.

Choosing not to nurse

A woman's choice regarding breastfeeding is influenced by many factors. Some of the suggested but not necessarily proven influences include the mother's satisfaction with the female role, her doctor's attitude toward breastfeeding, contentment with the shape of her body, attitudes toward the possibility of intellectual and creative stimulation during nursing, her work situation, and her ability to cope with feelings of asexuality, shame, and guilt. If a woman is prevented from breastfeeding despite her desire to do so because of reasons like illness, she is likely to

experience feelings of grief and loss, which can morph into feelings of anxiety, such as shame, anger, extended mourning, or depression.

Baby blues

The "baby blues" is a temporary psychological problem that many mothers briefly experience, commencing 3-5 days after delivery. Hormonal changes are likely the cause of "baby blues." The incidence of "baby blues" ranges by study, but more than half of new mothers report experiencing this phenomenon. "Baby blues" is characterized by changeable mood swings, tearfulness, headaches, irritability, inability to sleep, nightmares, alienation of others including the baby, and temporary cognitive problems. These mothers have transient shortfalls in cognitive function, in particular forgetfulness, which can be alleviated somewhat with analgesics. "Baby blues" is distinguished from postpartum depression or postpartum psychosis, both of which usually occur later, last longer and have more severe symptoms.

New mothers with mental illnesses

The postpartum period increases the risk of mental illness, and some mothers already have psychological problems that must be treated. The biggest issue is the choice of medication for these mental illnesses, particularly as it relates to passage into the milk and the amount that reaches the infant. For example, lithium (which is used to manage bipolar disorders) is considered acceptable during breastfeeding, but it does pass into breast milk and subsequently the child; hydration and monitoring of the infant is paramount. The sedative chlorpromazine, the anti-schizophrenic drug phenothiazine and the anti-depressant fluoxetine all pass into the breast milk but at levels that usually present no problem to the infant. One problem can be sudden weaning of depressed mothers from nursing which can bring on severe depression or attempts at suicide.

Postpartum depression

Postpartum depression generally occurs during the first year after delivery and lasts at least 2 weeks. It is not linked to feeding method and does occur in nursing mothers. Clinically severe depression can occur as early as 3 days after delivery but onset is usually later. Over half of women experiencing postpartum depression have some level of symptoms a year later. Investigations suggest that 10% or more of new mothers experience postpartum depression. Possible symptoms include tearfulness, sadness, anxiety, oversensitivity, and sleeplessness. The mother losses interest in external stimulation, she feels inadequate, and she may form suicidal tendencies. Triggers for postpartum depression include factors like hormone levels (high progesterone, low prolactin), a negative birth experience, or infants with disabilities or other problems.

Possible effects on infant

Maternal postpartum depression can negatively impact the emotional and cognitive progress of the infant. This occurs because the mother typically does not respond to infant cues and requirements. She often fails at breastfeeding for a variety of reasons, including a lack of satisfaction and joy from the act of nursing and a failure to understand the somatic nature of her difficulties. Her distraction from the child is compounded by her sense of isolation and lack of support. Poor motor scores and high irritability in infants at age 8 weeks correlate with maternal depression. Babies of depressed mothers cry more. Studies have also shown that children born to mothers who experience postpartum depression have a greater incidence of behavioral problems up to at least age 6.

Postpartum psychosis

During the postpartum period, about 0.1%-0.2% of mothers experience some sort of psychiatric disorder, and the risk of a serious psychiatric illness increases 15-fold after childbirth. At least half of these health problems are considered affective disorders, which are prolonged emotional disturbances or depression. Postpartum psychosis can also manifest as schizophrenia, organic psychiatric illnesses, and anxiety disorders. It typically occurs within 2-4 weeks after delivery, but can start as late as 8 weeks postpartum and last for different lengths of time depending on the diagnosis. Women with postpartum psychosis can have either heightened or diminished motor activity and significant mood deviations. They many experience hallucinations, confusion, severe depression (generally called postpartum depression), and/or mania.

Edinburgh Postnatal Depression Scale

The Edinburgh Postnatal Depression Scale (EPDS) is a series of 10 questions developed by the Department of Psychiatry at the University of Edinburgh. It is designed to be an adjunct to clinical diagnosis of postnatal or postpartum depression. The EPDS is usually administered to mothers 6-8 weeks after delivery. The mother underlines which answer of the possible 4 provided comes closest to her feelings. The questions address issues such as level of enjoyment, ability to laugh, feelings of blame, anxiety, panic, being overwhelmed, sleeplessness, sadness, crying, and thoughts of self-harm. Depending on the question, the response is scored from 0-3 points and a total of at least 12 or 13 points is considered suggestive of depression.

Effects of early maternal employment

Recent surveys show that in the United States, the rates of initiation of breastfeeding are at least as great in women who plan to return to work full- or part-time. A 2000 study by the Ross Products Division of Abbott Laboratories found that during the 6 months after delivery, part-time working mothers exhibit the highest rate of breastfeeding for all time points. Full-time work, outside the home does affect the duration of nursing and is correlated with earlier cessation of breastfeeding. At least half of previously employed new mothers return to work within 3 months of delivery and about 70% of mothers with children under 3 years old are employed full-time. Working mothers are motivated by diverse factors, such as needed income and personal fulfillment. Other factors such as family stability and quality time spent with the child affect young children at least as much as the status of maternal employment.

Factors influencing continued breastfeeding

In order to combine work outside the home and breastfeeding, the mother must be able to nurse, pump, or manually-express milk and store it at her place of employment. Certain types of jobs facilitate this more easily, and, therefore, enhance the probability breastfeeding longer. Cottage industries and workplaces that provide childcare or designated private areas for expression and milk storage actual nursing encourage continued breastfeeding. Some companies do not permit mothers to nurse or do not have formal breastfeeding policies or facilities. Maternal absenteeism correlates to feeding method; studies have shown that breastfeeding reduces absenteeism. Fatigue and sleep deprivation are hallmarks for all new mothers and can be accentuated when returning to work.

Maintaining an adequate milk supply while working is difficult and may contribute to a mother's decision to wean.

Counseling for working mothers wishing to breastfeed

Mothers often have unrealistic expectations about parenting, the fatigue associated with being a new mother, and working. Health care professionals should counsel new and expectant mothers with regard to childcare, time management, availability of facilities to pump and store milk at work, and parenting issues relevant to working mothers.

Breastfeeding mothers should also be counseled with regard to introducing a bottle to the infant, which usually occurs at least 10 days prior to the return to work. The child may not readily accept bottle-feeding so exercises to encourage it may be necessary, including tactics like warming the milk, creating a soothing environment, isolating the mother from the area, using a soft nipple and small bottle initially, and feeding in a position similar to nursing. The mother is generally encouraged to have the caregiver feed the child solid foods after 6 months of age to supplement breastfeeding.

Infant illness and relationship to daycare

Young children in daycare have increased rates of illness, including hepatitis A, meningitis, and diarrhea. There is evidence that they also experience more otitis media, respiratory illness, and cytomegalovirus infections. These increased infectivity rates extend to people with whom they are in contact, such as the family, other household contacts, and their daycare teachers. Therefore, if the child is in daycare, the facility should be carefully scrutinized in terms of healthy procedures, policies toward breastfeeding, and provisions for storage of breast milk. The latter two points are important because of the protective effects of breast milk, especially during the first 6 months of life. Breast milk can withstand longer storage at room temperature, can be used again, and contains antibodies and other protective factors; formula always has to be refrigerated and must be thrown out if feeding is unsuccessful.

Mother support groups

The major mother support groups include:

- La Leche League - Founded in Illinois, in 1957, it now has about 3000 groups in 66 countries, has published several editions of *The Womanly Art of Breastfeeding*, provides instructional classes and telephone counselors that provide support, and direct women to appropriate local physicians and resources.
- International Childbirth Education Association - Available in many countries, takes a family and complete child birthing approach to education and support.
- Breastfeeding Association of South Africa - Voluntary association independent of the government. This group addresses a variety of issues ranging from infertility to loss of a child.
- Ammehjelpen International Group – A Norwegian support group.
- Nursing Mothers' Association – An Australian support group.
- National Childbirth Trust – A British support group.

Studies indicate that mothers attending support groups tend to maintain breastfeeding longer.

Doula

A *doula* is a trained person who provides physical, emotional, and educational support to a mother prior to, during, and after childbirth. In more traditional cultures, a doula is often available to facilitate the period of transition or rite of passage called birth and motherhood. This period is called matrescence, and these cultural systems place an emphasis on the mother's comfort during this time. In today's society, however, most mothers are relatively isolated within the nuclear family and do not have a doula. These cultural shifts make other resources such as support groups and community services increasingly important for the adjustment of new mothers.

Breastfeeding support organizations

Organizations that promote and support breastfeeding include:

- United States Breastfeeding Committee (USBC) - A joint partnership of a number of organizations, including the American Academy of Pediatrics, the American College of Obstetricians and Gynecologists, and La Leche League International; also includes participation of government bureaus, such as the National Institutes of Health.
- Wellstart International – A private group that works in conjunction with the U. S. Agency for International Development (AID) and others to educate health professionals regarding breastfeeding. Program offerings include Lactation Management Education (LME).
- Best Start – A private, non-profit group, primarily media-driven and concerned with social marketing approach; provides a

range of initiatives such as community networking and education (classes, activities), public service announcements, and development of products related to breastfeeding. Other organizations follow the Best Start model.

- Academy of Breastfeeding Medicine - International organization of physicians promoting their knowledge of the field and optimal practices in breastfeeding management.

There are many other government and private organizations concerned with promotion of breastfeeding.

Lactation consultant certification process

The La Leche League International developed the International Board of Lactation Consultant Examiners (IBLCE) as the credentialing organization for lactation consultants. The IBLCE certifies appropriate allied health professionals such as nurses, nurse practitioners, midwives, and sometimes dieticians or doctors who pass a written examination administered by the IBLCE. There are three pathways to certification culminating in the title of International Board Certified Lactation Consultant (IBCLC). Those are experience as lactation care provider, completion of an academic program, or through mentorship. The examination covers areas ranging from maternal and infant anatomy to pharmacology and ethical issues. It is given once a year and IBCLCs must recertify within 10 years. Another organization, the International Lactation Consultants Association (ILCA), has developed Standards of Practice for Lactation Consultants. The lactation consultant is an integral part of the healthcare team treating the new mother, especially in the days following delivery.

Peer counselors and peer support groups

A peer is a person of relatively equal standing in terms of age or social class. Peer counseling and support groups provided by various public health programs have been quite successful in guiding new mothers. Peer support is used in a variety of health care situations, such as for people with cancer or diabetes. In regards to childbearing, counselors who have been taught to provide multi-stage support for the woman through pregnancy, childbirth, and early child rearing (including breastfeeding) are most successful. For example, in the United States a program called Women, Infants, and Children (WIC) provides this type of counseling. Ideal peer counselors are lay employees who come from similar backgrounds to their target audience, practice good health procedures themselves, and are sympathetic and non-judgmental listeners. The peer counselor is not authorized to provide medical advice and should instruct the mother to seek medical care when appropriate.

Maternal and infant sleep patterns

New mothers generally experience sleep deprivation. During the first 24 hours after birth, neonates generally exhibit the following sleep pattern: alertness during the first 2 hours after birth, a light and deep sleep during the next 18 hours, and then growing wakefulness during hours 20-24. During the early weeks of life, the infant's sleep pattern is characterized by rapid eye movement or REM sleep, they have irregular heart and respiratory rates, and their body movements are very active. The proportion of REM sleep decreases and periods of quiet sleep increase at age 2-3 months. Thus, the mother has the opportunity for more sleep as well. Infants tend to be agitated and cry prior to sleeping as well as during

the periods of wakefulness between sleep.
Infants who are breastfed have been
found to wake more often at night and
have abbreviated sleep patterns relative
to those who are formula-fed.

Growth Parameters/Development

Parameters used to evaluate growth

The most commonly used growth parameters are weight and length, which many experts feel is a better criterion. Length and weight are not necessarily correlated. The knee to heel length, which increases in terms of percentage of total body length, is sometimes used. Another possible measurement is weight per unit of length. Gains in weight or length during selected time intervals may be used. Some authorities feel that head circumference, which correlates to brain growth, is important. Some anthropometric measurements like weight are deceptive; bottle-fed infants tend to gain more weight than those breastfed. But these infants do not necessarily gain greater length. Increased weight in bottle-fed infants may be due to overfeeding.

Standard anthropometric measurements and changes

Standard growth charts include mean weights (in grams) and lengths (in millimeters) for both males and females at certain time points. Other standard tables show mean weight gain (in g/day) and mean gain in length (in mm/day). The mean weight at various time points from 8-112 days is less for breastfed than formula-fed infants, and females tend to weigh less than their male counterparts. The nursing infants generally consume fewer calories by choice, but nutrition is adequate. The same patterns are seen to a much lower extent in mean length measurements; essentially length differs insignificantly between groups. Infants gain more weight and length on a daily basis between days 8 and 42 than they do between days 42 and 112. Boys generally gain more weight and length than girls during this time, and again the formula-fed children have slightly higher gains. Small-for-gestational age infants can experience accelerated catch-up growth if they are breastfed.

Effects of weaning to solids vs. prolonged breastfeeding

The timing of weaning to solid foods appears to influence growth. If a breastfed infant is weaned early, less than 6 months of age, some of their energy intake previously received from breast milk is supplanted by energy intake from the solid foods through the infant's own self-regulating mechanisms. For example, they may not eat all the food offered. Breastfed infants weaned between ages 4 and 7 months have consistently lower weight and weight per length measurements than those weaned later. The differences in growth do not appear to be related to protein intake, and human milk does not restrict growth. Various studies have found that infants who are exclusively breastfed much longer tend to be smaller; these findings may be biased by the fact that mothers with small infants may nurse longer.

Effects of breastfeeding on cognitive and motor development

Children who have been breastfed as infants average higher levels of cognition at age 7 as measured by tests for vocabulary, intelligence, and language development. Children in this age range also tend to have fewer conduct disorders. As they get older and grow into adolescence, previously breastfed children continue to perform slightly better than other groups in terms of cognitive and educational attainments. There is also some suggestion that breastfeeding high-risk infants can improve later measurements of intelligence. Some studies suggest that nursing enhances motor development as well. Isolated reports have shown improved speech patterns in previously breastfed 6 year olds (particularly boys) and increased visual acuity at 4 months in breastfed infants.

Associations between breastfeeding and obesity

In general, studies have found that new mothers who are obese have more difficulty initiating and continuing breastfeeding than normal weight women. Breastfed infants tend to be leaner than formula-fed babies. Studies suggest that breastfeeding coupled with late introduction of solid foods can help prevent infant obesity, lower their risk for respiratory and gastrointestinal diseases, and improve thyroid levels. Obese infants tend to lag in terms of development. Mean weight differences disappear as children get older. Most studies (human and animal) suggest that infant ingestion of species-specific milk reduces the possibility of obesity and high cholesterol levels in later life. Adults who were breastfed as infants generally have lower plasma cholesterol levels and less risk for heart disease.

BMI

BMI stands for body mass index which is defined as:
weight/(height)^2
If weight is expressed in kilograms, then height should be given in meters. Weight in pounds combined with height in inches can also be used. BMI measurements roughly classify individuals as underweight (BMI $\leq$ 19.8), normal (BMI 19.8 to 26.0), overweight (BMI 26.1 to 29.0), or obese (BMI > 29.0). BMI has significance in terms of defining the population at large and mothers before pregnancy. It can also be used for infants,

but other methods of evaluation are often used. Commonly the mean value + 2 standard deviations (SD) is used as a cutoff for obesity using factors like skin-fold thickness. Another definition of infant obesity is a specific low length combined with a particular high weight at different ages, using previously developed percentiles + 2 SD. The 85th percentile for weight versus length is a convenient cutoff. These latter types of measurements do not take into account variables like bone structure, and BMI is considered a better universal definition.

Preventing or diminishing unwanted infant weight gain

Excessive feeding should be terminated as it does not generally reflect nutritional needs. Exclusive breastfeeding should be used for 6 months. Instead of feeding the infant whenever they cry or express other needs, the mother should practice nonnutritive cuddling. The baby should be encouraged to be more active so as to use excess energy. This can be facilitated in young infants by use of less restrictive types of carriers and in older ones through play and crawling. If excessive growth continues, the mother's milk should be tested for hyperlipidemia using a creamatocrit, which is the percentage of cream as observed in a capillary tube. The fat and kilocalorie content of the milk should also be calculated.

Creamatocrit

A creamatocrit is a rapid way to determine fat, protein, and carbohydrate content of milk. It is often used to analyze milk in milk banks, but it is also indicated for mothers with suspected hyperlipidemia and obese infants. The mother's breast milk, generally fresh or fresh-frozen and thawed, is put in a hematocrit or capillary tube and spun in a centrifuge. The percentage of cream is the creamatocrit. The relationship between

- 91 -

creamatocrit and fat or kilocalorie content of the milk can be expressed as follows:

- Fat content (gm/L) = (creamatocrit percentage - 0.59)/0.146
- Energy content in kcal/L = 290 + (66.8 x creamatocrit percentage)

Other equations have also been developed.   A commercially available tool, the Creamatocrit Plus, is often utilized, which eliminates the need for calculations.

Premature infants

Gastrointestinal tract development and gastric emptying

Structurally, the gastrointestinal (GI) tract of the fetus progresses from formation of a primitive gut at 6-8 weeks in utero to a mature small intestine at 17-30 weeks. In the interim, the gut rotates, villi begin to protrude, cellular differentiation occurs, and digestive enzymes start to appear. Functionally, a swallow reflex begins as early as 15 weeks in utero and is followed by GI motor activity from week 23 on. Organized motility begins around week 28 followed by nutritive sucking and swallowing. The latter usually appears around week 32, but premature infants at a gestational age of 28 weeks, have been found to initiate breastfeeding. Premature infants will have slow gastric emptying unless they receive breast milk or certain compounds in their diet, such as starch. Breast-milk feedings enhance motility and stool passage, and half of the milk passes through the stomach within 25 minutes, while formulas (and other factors like illness) slow emptying to about 51 minutes.

Premature and low birth weight designations

An infant is said to be premature if they are less than 37 weeks of gestation at time of delivery. Low birth weight designations refer to weight cutoffs for infants, regardless of gestational age, although most of these babies are born prematurely. If an infant weighs less than 2500 g, they are of low birth weight (LBW). The cutoff for very low birth weight (VLBW) is below 1500 g, and premature infants with a radically low weight of less than 800 g are said to be of extremely low birth weight (ELBW). On the other hand, a full term baby who has a low birth weight is considered small-for-gestational-age (SGA).

Enteral feeding and breastfeeding

Enteral feeding triggers gut maturation in neonates through activation of gut peptides and hormones. Even very low birth weight (VLBW) preemies are used to swallowing up to 150 mL/kg/day of amniotic fluid in utero, which supplies protein needed after birth. VLBW infants have higher relative amounts of body water and muscle mass and lower amounts of fat reserves and glycogen stores. Their surface area is relatively high so they lose water through evaporation and need hydration. Premature infants consume relatively high amounts of oxygen due to high growth rates. They have a poor insulin response making them susceptible to hyperglycemia. All of these factors speak to the need for early enteral feedings. Human breast milk provides nutrients and enzymes that promote gut maturation of their immature GI tract and provides protection against infection. These infants usually require additional supplements to provide certain nutrients.

Recommendations for feeding

The beneficial effects of breastfeeding premature and low birth weight infants behoove the mother to begin milk expression, even if the baby is not ready to feed at the breast. Her colostrum can be given to the child initially via a gastric tube. A small, premature infant has limited caloric reserves relative to a larger preemie or full-term neonate. They also have a larger percentage of water and less protein, fat, and carbohydrate, which means they will starve without added calories. It is recommended that as soon as the infant can engage a nipple, breastfeeding is initiated. Not only does breast milk have protective effects, but it takes less energy for the baby to suckle at the breast (a normal response) than to drink from a bottle. Milk supply can be enhanced through techniques like use of a nursing supplementer, frequent pumping, warm soaks or massage of the breast, kangaroo care (maintaining skin-to-skin contact with the child), or pharmacologic stimulation. Infants are usually not discharged until they have persistent gains in weight, length, and head circumference and their biochemical profile is stable.

Optimal growth and protein requirements
Optimal growth expectations for premature infants are based on the standard growth curve, taking into account early gestation age. Bone mineral content (BMC) plotted against postnatal age and superimposed against the continued post conceptual age is used to generate a theoretical intrauterine BMC growth regression curve. Bone mineral content below the 95th percentile confidence limits of this curve suggests osteopenia. Protein requirements for premature, low birth weight infants are usually based on the child's birth weight. If they fall into the range of 800-1200 g at birth, their estimated requirements are 3.64 g/day with 4 g/day suggested. Premature infants who are larger at birth, 1200-1800 g, have estimated protein needs of 4.78 g/day, with 5.2 g/day suggested.

Low birth weight infants

Growth issues of VLBW infants
At the time of discharge, anthropometric measurements, such as head circumference, weight gain, or length, are not significantly different in breastfed or formula-fed groups regardless of birth weight. Later however, one of the major issues for VLBW infants is bone mineral content (BMC) and bone accretion. Premature babies often have reduced bone mineralization and inadequate levels of calcium and phosphorus, which can impede growth. Studies indicate that early fortification in conjunction with human milk contributes to greater BMC. These babies should receive stored milk (refrigerated or frozen) with added fortifier (100 mL/kg/day, if tolerated) until they are able to completely breastfeed or weigh in the range of 1800-2000 g. Fortifiers should contain multivitamins.

Iron deficiency is another concern in low birth weight infants who are breastfed. Iron supplementation beginning around 2 months or when birth weight doubles may be sufficient to protect against deficiency.

There is also anecdotal evidence that VLBW infants are more likely to develop hypertriglyceridemia if they are breastfed.

Breast milk supplementation
Low birth weight infants are generally premature, and the mother's breast milk often has deficiencies that must be supplemented with vitamins, minerals, and sometimes proteins, carbohydrates, or fat. Suggested vitamin supplementation includes: vitamin D (400 IU/day), vitamin A (1000-1500 IU/day), vitamin K (0.5-1.0 mg at birth, then 5 ug/kg/day), and vitamin E (25 IU/day initially, 5 IU/day after first month). Addition of other vitamins depends on individual circumstances. For example, vitamin C (up to 60 mg/day) should be supplemented if the child is receiving supplementary protein, and vitamin B_{12} is

- 93 -

indicated if the mother's diet is lacking it. Adequate mineral levels are important as well, and special attention should be paid to calcium and phosphorus to prevent rickets. Monitoring serum phosphorus and calcium via weekly assays may be necessary; phosphorus levels < 4 mg/dL require radiographs of the wrist. VLBW infants usually need copper supplementation during the first 3 months and iron fortification around age 2 months.

Brain growth and measures of
intelligence
At the time of their delivery, premature or low birth weight infants are in a period of rapid brain growth, which continues throughout the first year of their life. The nutrients that contribute to brain growth include taurine, cholesterol, omega-3 fatty acids, and amino sugars, all of which are found in human milk. A number of studies have shown the advantages of breastfeeding over regular or preterm formula in preterm infants in terms of intelligence, cognition, motor skills, and visual acuity. Time points of measurement have ranged from age 3 months to 8 years. Moreover, partial breast milk intake has a positive effect on the neurodevelopment of a child. The effects of fortification on neurodevelopment are unclear; at least one study failed to show neurodevelopment effects of fortification at 18 months. Formula-fed preemies are much more prone to retinopathy than those who are breastfed.

Digestion and absorption of premature and term neonates

Developmental markers and enzymes associated with the gastrointestinal tract appear at various time points during gestation. For example, some enzymes, such as lactase and dipeptidases, are found as early as 10 weeks; developmental markers in the colon and stomach appear at week 20; and squamous cells are not observed in the esophagus until week 28. Functionally, a mouthing type of suckling occurs at week 24 and immature sucking and swallowing appear at week 26. The ability of a neonate to digest and absorb proteins, fats, and carbohydrates is dependent on the availability of certain enzymes and transport mechanisms. Full-term newborns have complete or detectable levels of important enzymes as well as uptake and absorption mechanisms, but depending on the week of gestation at birth, premature infants may not. Therefore, certain nutrients may not be tolerated by the preterm infant.

Lactoengineering

Lactoengineering is the manipulation of human donor milk to produce specific human milk nutrients. Typical procedures include separation of cream and protein portions, reduction of lactose levels, and use of high-temperature short-time (HTST) pasteurization. Protein or triglycerides obtained through lactoengineering are then used to supplement the mother's own milk or pooled human milk. There is evidence that addition of protein does improve weight gain and length, and premature infants at birth have low levels of true protein. The benefits of fat supplementation are unclear, however. In addition, similar attempts to engineer cow's milk for added protein have not yet shown distinct advantages.

Fortified human milk

There are a number of commercially available human milk fortifiers. Powdered supplements, such as Enfamil and Similac fortifiers, are meant to add nutrients to a mother's or pooled donor human milk. Fortified human milk has been shown to increase weight gain, length, head circumference, bone mineral content, and measurements related to protein, such as nitrogen balance and BUN. Fortifiers do not enhance host defense mechanisms, diminish enter colitis related to infection, or improve feeding tolerance. They do supply additional energy and usually extra carbohydrate, protein, calcium, phosphorus, magnesium, sodium, zinc, copper, and vitamins. Fortifiers do not interfere with the protective effects of human milk unless iron is added, hence the recommendation to hold iron supplementation until the infant's birth weight doubles.

Preterm and term colostrum

The colostrum of a mother delivering preterm has significantly higher levels of the immunoglobulins of the IgA class (particularly secretory IgA) and the proteins lysozyme and lactoferrin than that of term colostrum. These high concentrations help protect the premature infant from infections. Morbidity and death from necrotizing enterocolitis (NEC) is of great concern in premature and other high-risk neonates. NEC is significantly more prevalent in formula-fed than breastfed infants delivered at gestational age of 27 weeks or less. Preterm infants who receive breast milk have less hospital-acquired infections, incidence of sepsis, and fewer upper respiratory infections during the first year of life.

Associated problems with SGA infants

A small-for-gestational-age (SGA) infant is one born full-term but with low birth weight (<10th percentile). They also tend to be undersized in terms of length and head circumference. SGA babies usually have low calcium levels, which can be rectified with early use of breast milk. They are often hypoglycemic due to suppressed glycogen stores and may experience hypothermia shortly after birth. An SGA child usually has an immature gut, a poor suck, and poor synchronization of sucking and swallowing. Their neurodevelopment can be retarded, but breastfeeding has been found to improve later measures of mental status.

Infant development and weaning

Weaning is the introduction of foods in addition to breast milk in an infant's diet. Weaning is usually initiated gradually and led by the child, although the time of weaning is often culturally determined. Attainment of certain developmental milestones also plays a role. Milestones that affect nutritional needs in the infant are important markers to begin weaning. For example, additional iron requirements at 6 months and protein needs at 9 months are addressed by addition of solid foods. Solids can only be introduced after the child has cultivated the chew-swallow reflex, which can begin as early as 4 months but is not fully developed for several more months. If the infant is not given solid foods around this time, they may be poor chewers. Breastfed infants are susceptible to weaning at age 6 months (the recommended age by many organizations) due to the aforementioned reasons, greater exposure to a variety of tastes, and other social/cultural influences.

Problems associated with weaning

The most prevalent weaning concern is weaning diarrhea, which due to the loss of breast milk protective factors reactions to newly introduced foods. In underdeveloped countries, malnutrition is an issue upon weaning, and infant mortality rates increase. A mother may have to initiate abrupt or emergency weaning because of serious illness or unexpected separation. She may develop milk fever (a brief bout of fever, chills, and dejection), engorgement, and depression due to abrupt hormonal (prolactin) changes. Conversely, breastfed infants may initiate transient nursing strikes or refuse to nurse, the causes of which may be maternal (changes in menstruation or diet) or infant (teething or an earache). Usually breastfeeding can be resumed if the child is cuddled and quieted.

Interpretation of Research

Theories applied to lactation practice

A theory is a hypothetical or speculative, rather than an empirical or completely fact-driven view of a situation. A theoretical model or framework is a depiction of concepts from a theory as they relate to a particular study. The following theories are some of those used in lactation practice and research design.

- Maternal Role Attainment Theory (Rubin, Mercer and Ferketich) - Holds that maternal role is attained by letting go of old roles, having experiences associated with being a mother (such as successful breastfeeding), and identification with the infant.
- Bonding and Attachment Theory (Klaus and Kennel) - Claims that close contact between parent and infant shortly after birth enhances optimal child development; later attachment is also influential and necessary due to the malleability of humans.
- Darwinian Medicine - Adaptation of Darwin's theory of natural selection and evolution to human diseases; relevance to lactation practice includes practices that are protective mechanisms, such as frequent nightly interactions between co-sleeping mother and child to prevent SIDS.
- Self-Care Theory -Self-care activities are those done on an individual basis to promote health and well-being; used in lactation practice to encourage mother and family to use their means toward providing a favorable breastfeeding experience.
- Self-Efficacy Theory (Bandura) - Theorizes that people learn to execute certain tasks based on their own perceptions about their abilities; perceptions are affected by internal motivation, emotions, and the environment. This theory has been used in lactation practice to develop task-oriented scales to predict breastfeeding patterns.
- Theory of Planned Behavior (TPB) and Theory of Reasoned Action (TRA) - Both based on assumptions that behavior is influenced by the intention to perform that behavior; both theories include personal intention and perceptions relative to social norms and TPB also includes the ease of performance (control). These theories have been used to predict breastfeeding success.

Parent-child interaction model and the Child Health Assessment Interaction Model

The parent-child or caregiver-infant interaction model asserts that certain personal characteristics of the dyad determine the degree of positive interaction. For the mother, these characteristics include being able to sense infant cues, taking action when the child is suffering, and using tactics that encourage growth experiences for the baby. For the child, traits include the abilities to give clear cues and respond to the parent.

The Child Health Assessment Interaction Model is a theoretical framework that utilizes the above concepts. It is illustrated by three overlapping circles, the largest being the mother, followed by the environment and the infant. Each circle of influence includes factors that enhance the interactions between mother, child, and environment.

Qualitative research methods

Qualitative research methods take a humanistic approach and are predominant in the social sciences. Some of the most frequently used methods are described here:

- Phenomenology is a method that strives to combine scientific and humanistic approaches. It uses participant descriptions of life experiences to elucidate their fundamental nature.
- Ethnography is a methodology aimed at discovering cultural beliefs and practices through examination of the views of individuals in the cultural group.
- Grounded theory constructs a theoretical framework based on actual data collected from population groups.
- Discourse analysis looks at language and ways of communicating in order to disclose core tenets.

Quantitative research methods

Quantitative research methods attempt to find measurable ways to describe situations through either non-experimental or experimental studies. There are two approaches to quantitative non-experimental research, descriptive or correlational studies. Descriptive studies are generally used to glean information in areas of minimal knowledge. Correlational studies look at the connection between two or more factors and determine whether trends are statistically significant. Data is collected in a very controlled manner in correlational studies.

Experimental studies are controlled and designed to determine possible cause and effect. A proper experimental study is characterized by rigorous control of the experimental circumstances, administration of a prescribed experimental intervention by an investigator, and randomization of experimental and control groups. The experimental circumstances or treatments are considered the independent variable. If one of the criteria for a true experimental study cannot be met exactly, perhaps due to ethical concerns, the research method is quasi-experimental.

Other research methods

Many studies combine both qualitative and quantitative research methods. In addition, there are other techniques utilized. Observational research is often used to characterize animal or human behavioral patterns. Variations of observational research are ethology, the study of animals (or humans) in their natural habitat, and behavioristic psychology, a non-analytic approach emphasizing observation, measurement, and modification of behavior. Historical research compiles previous observations on a subject in an attempt to find common trends. Some research methods have a social agenda. These include research conducted from a feminist perspective and participatory action. Participatory action refers to an interactive type of research project directed towards positive change.

Fundamentals of research projects

All research projects should incorporate certain fundamentals in terms of their design. These fundamentals should be included in research proposals, reports, and articles written about the work. They should also be adhered to during conduct of the research and considered when one is evaluating other's work. The first part of any research project is definition of the research problem and identification of the purpose of the study. A review of previous literature on the subject is essential before beginning the study and should be referenced. The literature review is a starting point to pose a question and is more rigorously used for research design in quantitative studies. Provisions for the protection of human subjects must be included. Suitable research methods and type of data analysis must be selected before study commencement. Results, conclusions, and discussion should be based the observations.

Research problems and project purpose

The research problem and purpose of a potential study are usually posed as either a relevant question or a declarative statement. The mode and range of scope may depend on the depth of current knowledge about the topic and the research method to be used. For example, topics where less is known lend themselves to broader questions and qualitative methods. Themes where there is greater knowledge usually call for more focused questions and quantitative methods. The researcher should also consider whether the problem can be approached scientifically by evaluating certain factors. These include the appropriateness of the research design to the expressed problem; the availability of study participants; study feasibility in terms of time, money, and equipment; and ability to adhere to ethical requirements.

Variables in research study design

A variable is something that can change or vary. In quantitative or experimental research projects, variables are typically some type of characteristic that can be controlled or measured. There is at least one independent variable that the investigator can theoretically control, and at least one dependent, or outcome variable that is influenced by the independent variable. The research is aimed at understanding the relationship between the two variables. A characteristic research design would be using a population with similar traits (the independent variable) and randomly assigning those to experimental versus control (untreated) groups in order to examine the differences in outcome (the dependent variable). There may be confounding variables that influence the outcome as well. Qualitative studies are more likely to look for relationships in a less critical manner.

Hypothesis

A hypothesis is a formal declaration of the relationship between two or more variables in a study population. Qualitative studies can engender hypotheses. Quantitative studies, particularly experimental research projects, generally have predicted hypotheses that they test by examining the relationships among variables using data analysis and statistics. The research may use a hypothesis written in null form (in other words, a presumption of no difference between groups) that if disproved statistically implies a true difference. Correlational studies usually form hypotheses that look at general relationships, such as positive effects.

Operational definitions

It is imperative to include extremely clear operational definitions when designing a credible research study. Particularly in experimental studies, the independent variable (often the study population) and the intervention regimen(s) must be defined in a manner that is incontrovertible. For example, in studies about breastfeeding, the investigator must be explicit about defining breastfeeding categories (such as timing, type and number of alternate feedings, premature versus term birth, etc.). The clarity of operational definitions affects sample size of the independent variables or groups, the ability to collect data, the accuracy of data analysis, the outcomes, and the interpretation of the data.

Rights of human subjects in research studies

All research studies done on human subjects should preserve certain rights of the subject. The study design should include provisions against any risk of harm; complete disclosure about the intent of the study, procedures, and time involved; the guarantee that refusal to participate or withdrawal from the study is acceptable and will not affect care; and means of protecting the privacy and confidentiality of the subject at all times. Most research studies are performed under the auspices of institutions, like health care facilities or universities, which have established ethical review boards to screen research proposals. In addition, an informed consent form outlining all of the above factors must be freely signed by any individual (or their representative) undergoing clinical trials.

Methods outlined in research proposals

Research study methods should include clear descriptions of the setting, the target population to be studied, the sampling process, the methods of data collection, and the approaches to data analysis. The setting is either the location of study or the resources for recruiting subjects. The target population cannot generally be examined in its entirety, which means some sort of sampling process is necessary for subject selection. Sampling methods are both random in nature and based on probability or they are nonrandom and non-probability based (discussed further elsewhere). The data collection method should be suitable to the research method and population

being studied. For breastfeeding research, self-report questionnaires, interviews, or observations are often used, but they must be designed to ensure maximum participation and precise information. Biophysical measurements, such as head circumference, heart rates, prolactin levels, and milk composition can also be utilized. Data analysis methods are very dependent on other aspects of design.

Sampling methods

Researchers select samples or subjects from a larger population group. This sampling can be based on probability or non-probability criteria. Probability sampling is preferable for quantitative studies because it is more representative of the target population. Subjects are randomly chosen from a larger group through simple, systematic, or stratified random sampling. Simple random sampling employs completely unbiased means, such as using a random sampling table, tossing a coin, or picking numbers from a hat. Selecting individuals at certain intervals from a completely random list is systematic sampling. Stratified random sampling picks subjects based on known distributions of subgroups in a populace. Research projects involving humans often cannot identify all appropriate subjects necessitating non-probability sampling. Types of non-probability sampling include convenience sampling from an easily available source; network sampling (also called nominated or snowball sampling), which uses people in the study to identify other potential participants; solicited volunteer sampling, which uses advertising; purposeful sampling; and theoretical sampling.

Methods employed in qualitative research

Qualitative studies tend to use non-probability methods of population sampling and have relatively small numbers of subjects (up to about 50). The number and type of subjects may be somewhat open-ended. Theoretical sampling, in which initial participants are selected by a non-probability method but later subjects are chosen based on growing knowledge, is often employed. The means of data collection are usually document examinations, interviews, field observations, and focus groups. Data analysis is generally a continuous and growing process. Different types of qualitative research tend to rely on particular types of data analysis. For example, phenomenological studies often use techniques like identification of common themes and development of structural descriptions of experiences from the participants' point of view. Ethnographic analysis usually describes social and cultural patterns (descriptive) or examines the meanings and preconceptions associated with actions in cultural groups (analytical). In grounded theory based projects, data is analyzed in a more structured fashion though use of coding and categorization.

Reliability of qualitative research

Qualitative research is inherently less reproducible and reliable than quantitative research. Qualitative research can be considered relatively reliable if it meets 4 criteria. The first is its credibility or believability. Credibility is enhanced by incorporation of study design features such as long periods of data collection, use of several data sources, peer review, and informed participant involvement. Another measure of reliability is dependability or trustworthiness, which can generally be improved by having another researcher review the analysis. Ability to confirm the data is also important. Lastly, a study is considered more reliable if its observations can be transferred to other groups or settings.

Sampling and data collection in quantitative research studies

Determination of appropriate sample size for quantitative research studies depends on factors such as the type of investigation, subject availability, funding, and length of the study. In general, the sample size should be as large as possible, especially for correlational studies. Statisticians or computer programs can approximate a suitable sample size. The participants should be randomly assigned to experimental or control groups for purposes of fairness and non-bias. Epidemiological studies, which look at patterns of disease development, are specialized types of quantitative surveys. They are generally done retrospectively as case-control studies, in which subjects are weighed against a control group, or cohort studies, in which individuals exposed or not subject to potential risk factors are followed over time. Data collection for quantitative studies, as for others, must be carefully controlled. The added dimension in data collection is that for correlational and any type of experimental study; statistical analysis is only possible if data can be condensed into some type of numerical connotation.

Reliability in data collection
Reliability and validity are essential to quantitative research studies. Reliability refers to the exactness and consistency of data collection and assessment tools. There are several important components of reliability. One is interrater reliability, which is the accurateness and constancy of data collection. Interrater reliability is enhanced by using the same machinery or observers throughout the study.

Another aspect is intrarater reliability, the exactness over time.
There is also test-retest reliability, which refers to agreement of measurements at two different time points. In this case, the two measurements may have a high

degree of correlation or if an event has occurred (such as postpartum depression in the interim), one may be much lower. To be considered reliable, a study should also have internal consistency, which generally refers to the statistical agreement in the way individuals answer related questions. It is often determined using Cronbach's alpha, a type of reliability coefficient.

<u>Validity in data collection</u>

Validity refers to how logical and meaningful the method of data collection is relative to the underlying hypothesis. There are 4 components of validity that might be used. Content validity, which means that relevant questions are asked, is essential for descriptive studies. Another component is concurrent validity, or the degree of equivalence between similar assessment tools. Construct validity refers to whether the means of assessment actually quantify the intended measurement. Some tools also have predictive validity, which means they are designed to determine future outcomes based on current measurements. Commonly used breastfeeding assessment tools that have some built-in predictive validity include the Breastfeeding Attrition Prediction Tool (BABT), the Maternal Breastfeeding Evaluation Scale (MBFES), and the Breastfeeding Self-Efficacy Scale (BSES).

Breastfeeding assessment tools and questionnaires

The most commonly used breastfeeding assessment tools and questionnaires are:
- Breastfeeding Attrition Prediction Tool (BAPT) - Pinpoints women who may wean early through measurement of 4 factors; reliable by Cronbach's alphas, has prediction validity.
- Maternal Breastfeeding Evaluation Scale (MBFES) -

Intended to evaluate complete breastfeeding experience of the mother, uses a 30-point Likert scale, evaluates areas like role attainment and infant satisfaction, acceptable reliability by Cronbach's alphas and test-retest correlation coefficients, and also has predictive validity.
- Breastfeeding Self-Efficacy Scale (BSES) - Evaluates the confidence level of nursing mothers by looking at various skills and beliefs, very high reliability using Cronbach's alpha, and possesses validity in terms of content and prediction of feeding method.
- LATCH Breastfeeding Assessment Tool - Uses parameters such as latch-on and perceptible swallowing to determine effectiveness of breastfeeding during first week after delivery; it is less well-characterized but has shown interrater reliability.
- Infant Breastfeeding Assessment Tool - Evaluates breastfeeding ability with 4 scales, has interrater reliability, and content validity.

Levels of data measurement

Quantitative studies require numerical analysis of data. The data can be measured at a nominal, ordinal, or interval/ratio level. Nominal measurements are those in which data points are placed into discrete but unordered categories; they are appropriate for descriptive studies. Ordinal measurements consign ranked data categories with disparate intervals. For example, a multipoint Likert scale, which measures the extent of agreement or disagreement with a statement, or the scales used by common breastfeeding assessment tools are ordinal measurements. Data points that are ordered and linear are interval/ratio measurements. These include measurements such as blood pressure, weight, and duration of breastfeeding, if clearly defined. Ordinal and interval/ratio measurements are more applicable to correlational and experimental studies.

Parametric and nonparametric statistical methods

Parametric statistical methods are more critical types of analysis than nonparametric procedures and are only appropriate for correlational, experimental, or quasi-experimental studies. They should only be used when there has been random sample selection, a normal distribution of variables between research groups, and quantification of the dependent variable(s) is expressed at the interval/ratio level.

Nonparametric statistical methods are those that have no underlying assumptions about distribution. They are used for smaller sample populations where characteristics are unknown and the level of quantification is only at the nominal or ordinal level. Nonparametric tests can be used for any type of quantitative study, depending on the specific test. They are appropriate for descriptive studies, which cannot be analyzed using parametric methods.

Statistical parameters used in correlational studies

Correlational studies are often expressed by some of the following terms:
- Correlation coefficient - The degree of correlation between two variables indicating whether or not they have a relationship; values range from +1 (strong positive relationship) to -1 (strong negative relationship)

with values near 0 demonstrating absence of a link.
- Risk ratio (RR, also known as relative risk) - Used in cohort studies to represent the frequency of disease or condition in exposed group relative to rate in unexposed control group; expressed as: RR = % positive in exposed group/% positive in control group = $[a/(a+b)]/[c/(c+d)]$, where a = positive cases in exposed group, b = negative cases in exposed group, c = positive cases in control group, and d= negative cases in control group.
- Odds ratio (OR) - Used in case studies with same types of variables as risk ratio; ratio of chance of exposure in cases relative to controls; OR = ad/bc.
- High risk or odds ratios greater than 1.0 are suggestive of increased risk in exposed group, low ones indicate decreased risk.
- There are also ordinal tests that are used to examine data, including Spearman's Rho test, Kendall's Tau test, and the parametric Pearson-r test.

Statistical parameters used in experimental studies

Experimental studies are often expressed by some of the following terms:
- p-value - Reflection of the probability or mathematical likelihood of an event, used to express statistical significance of results and whether or not the null hypothesis (which would mean no difference between groups) should be rejected; most common p-value selected is .05, or a 5 in 100 chance of error.
- Multivariate analysis - Simultaneous analysis of at least 3

variables through advanced techniques, such as multiple regressions, analysis of covariance (ANCOVA), and multivariate analysis of variance (MANOVA).

- t-test - Interval parametric test using relatively small sample to test for distribution in larger populations; has two forms, the pooled t-test for two independent groups, and the paired t-test for two dependent or paired groups f-test or ANOVA - Analysis of variance or difference in outcomes to determine contributing factors; interval parametric test for two or more experimental groups.

A number of non-parametric tests are also used, in particular chi-square variations.

Statistics used for descriptive studies

For the most part, data from descriptive studies should be collected in nominal or ordinal nonparametric measurements. If there is only one variable in the study, the commonly used statistical representations are frequency; percentage or proportion; mode, the value that occurs most frequently; median, or the middle value in a set of ordered values; mean, the average value; and standard deviation (SD), a statistical measurement of deviation from the mean. The latter two statistical parameters can only be used if the there is an interval or linear relationship with quantifiable data points. In studies with two or more variables, data might be expressed by a contingency table, cross tabulation, or chi-square.

Guidelines for evaluation of research studies

Clinicians must be able to evaluate research studies. A good study has a clearly elucidated and scientifically sound statement of the problem and purpose. A review of the literature should be included, and gaps of knowledge should be indicated. Human rights protections should be outlined. The research design, sampling procedures, and techniques used for data collection and analysis should be appropriate to the project and clearly stated in the research paper. The article should include a results section. If the study is qualitative, this is where actual descriptive narratives are included. If the study is quantitative in nature, then data should be expressed as tables or graphs using appropriate statistical analysis, and outlier observations should be noted without bias. There should also be a discussion section in which the investigator interprets the data internally and relative to outside findings. Conclusions about the study should be given succinctly. Often the potential clinical importance is included.

Evidence-based medicine and nursing

Evidence-based medicine (EBM) is the incorporation of practices into health care that have been shown by research to be useful. It implies that the health professional is cognizant of current research data, in particular randomized clinical trials. EBM is considered to be the highest standard of clinical care. By definition, EBM only utilizes information from research that is experimental and scientific in nature. Evidence-based nursing (EBN) is an extension of EBM used by the nursing community and experts such as lactation consultants. In addition to studies that are more quantitative, EBN incorporates other findings that are relevant and of benefit.

Perspectives used for health care research

A positivist perspective is one in which every attempt is made to use methods and reach conclusions that are based on objectivity, quantitative measurement, and non-biased observations. Strict positivism relies on traditional quantitative methods. A more adaptable version of positivism, which also happens to be the dominant worldview currently used in research, is postpositive perspective, in which approximations such as probability are acceptable as well. Qualitative research usually uses a naturalistic or humanistic perspective. Here phenomena are described in detail and theories are spawned through inductive reasoning of developing ideas. A critical or emancipatory perspective combines several types of perspectives, usually postpositivist, humanistic, and cultural influences. An emancipatory perspective is generally used to stimulate social change, and it is commonly used in areas like feminist or minority group research.

Ethical and Legal Issues

IBLCE Code of Ethics

General principles

A code of ethics is a system of moral principles that governs the conduct of a person or a particular group. The IBLCE has embraced 25 principles of ethical practice for an International Board Certified Lactation Consultant (IBCLC). Some are universal moral codes about provision of professional services that are objective and respectful, without conflict of interest, performed without discrimination, done in good faith with integrity and evenhandedness, and based on current and scientific principles. The Code of Ethics also addresses issues like maintaining confidentiality, being accountable for one's own actions, providing clients with sufficient information to make informed decisions (including products used), and seeking referrals for issues outside their realm of knowledge. Several of the principles talk about truth in advertising services or any conflicts of interest. The Code also addresses refusal of favors from patients, the need to obtain consent from the mother when using any type of media recording for professional purposes, recognition of intellectual property rights, and the obligation to withdraw services if the professional engages in substance abuse or becomes disabled in a way that affects their provision of care.

Principles specific to the profession

Among the 25 principles espoused in the IBLCE Code of Ethics, several are specific to the profession. These include #14, which addresses truthful representation about current IBCLC certification and the possibility of disciplinary action if misrepresented. This is taken further in principle #21, which requires submission to disciplinary action if convicted of a felony or misdemeanor, if restricted by state or local government for violation of one of the principles of the Code, if a governmental or licensing body determines malfeasance, or simply if a principle of the Code was violated. Principles #22 and #24, respectively, require the consultant to uphold the Code of Ethics for International Board Certified Lactation Consultants and the International Code of Marketing of Breast-Milk Substitutes.

ILCA Standards of Practice

All IBCLCs should adhere to the International Lactation Consultant Association's (ILCA) *Standards of Practice for International Board Certified Lactation Consultants.* There are 4 standards and subdivisions within each.

Standard 1: Professional Responsibilities - This has 8 subdivisions, some of which address adherence to ILCA Standards of Practice, IBLCE Code of Ethics, World Health Assembly resolutions, and the International Code of Marketing Breast-Milk Substitutes. Professional responsibilities also include being aware of conflicts of interest, advocating for breastfeeding, promoting the mother-child nursing relationship, and maintaining knowledge and certification through continuing education, periodic evaluation, and support of lactation research.

Standard 2: Legal Considerations - This standard concerns IBCLCs' contract to practice within their local legal constraints. There are 5 subdivisions which address the issues of working within the institutional policies of their employer (or clearly stated policies if self-employed), transparency regarding fees before provision of care, obtaining informed consent, protection of client confidentiality, and maintenance of records.

ILCA Standard 3: Clinical Practice has 4 subdivisions and addresses provision of clinical lactation care within the context of an interactive health care team. Section 3.1, "Assessment," addresses assessment through use of a clinical history of mother and infant, objective and subjective data, and discussion. Then section 3.2, "Plan" discusses analysis of the above data, development of a care plan, and follow-up arrangements. The bulk of this standard is devoted to section 3.3, "Implementation." This section enumerates factors needed for clinical implementation of the plan, such as techniques that accommodate the mother; translation if appropriate; use of healthy, safe, and universal precautions; use of oral or written instructions and demonstrations; provision of referrals if necessary; utilization of appropriate and well-maintained equipment and explanation of such to the client; and documentation to be shared with other members of the health care team. Lastly, section 3.4, "Evaluation" talks about the need to evaluate results and change the care plan if necessary.

ILCA Standard 4: Breastfeeding Education and Counseling discusses the importance of the educational and counseling aspects of IBCLC care. There are 5 subsections to standard 4. The first 4 subsections are about the lactation consultant's interaction with the mother. They discuss education of the parent and other family members to promote informed decisions, being sensitive to the mother's concern's and practical ways to approach them, providing information that will promote the most favorable nursing practices and minimize problems, and giving emotional support and positive reinforcement. Section 4.5 states that evidence-based information and clinical skills should be communicated to other health care providers involved.

Scope of practice

The IBLCE has developed a framework for the Scope of Practice for International Board Certified Lactation Consultants. The underlying tenet of this document is capable, evidence-based care. It states that IBCLCs are duty-bound to uphold professional standards, promote and support breastfeeding, provide expert services for the mother and family, maintain records and report results to all involved, protect the privacy and confidentially of all parties, and proceed with reasonable diligence. Many of the components of the scope of practice are outlined further elsewhere in discussions about ILCA Standards of Practice and IBLCE Code of Ethics, which combined address the vast majority of issues covered by the Scope of Practice.

Charting and report writing

Lactation consultants must chart each exchange that they have with the mother and infant. This documentation provides information to other health care workers, shows that quality care was provided, authenticates insurance claims, and can serve as legal evidence. The data provided may also be used for research purposes. There are two types of charting, narrative and problem-oriented. Narrative charting uses diary-type documentation in which a date and time is noted and then a progress note is added. Today charting is more often problem-oriented. This is a more ordered format. The most common form of problem-oriented charting documents six parameters: available subjective data (S), objective data (O), an assessment and nursing diagnosis based on these (A), a care plan (P) originating from these data and assessments, subsequent or intended interventions (I), and an evaluation (E) of outcomes.

Clinical care plans

Clinical care plans for each patient are obligatory in hospital settings per the Joint Commission on Accreditation of Health care Organizations (JCAHO) and are also required legally for practice. Depending on the circumstances, a custom-developed individual care plan or a standard published care plan appropriate for use with similar cases may be used. For both, intended interventional activities are listed and the date they are performed is typically recorded. A widely used type of clinical care plan is the development of a critical care path or clinical path that indicates important steps in the process.

Legal terms applicable to lactation consultant practice

"Battery" is the unlawful use of force on someone. The term applies to any situation in which there is offensive touching without the other person's consent. As applied to lactation consultant practice, this definition might extend to any circumstances where a mother or infant is touched, and as such, prior verbal and (preferably) written permission should be obtained. Other potentially legal situations include the infliction of emotional distress (through reckless acts or remarks) and the breach of warranty (non-provision of promised services). A tort is a civil wrongdoing for which damages may be solicited; this term often applies if confidentiality has been breached. Patient records are admissible legal documentation. Generally a lactation consultant is protected from the expense of liability through institutional or office "umbrella" insurance. Those in private practice should maintain some level of private insurance.

Reimbursement procedures for services in U.S.

In hospital and similar settings, lactation consultants (LC) may be salaried and their services (possibly including a postpartum visit) are contracted through a third-party payer as a percentage of total maternity care. In the United States, the third-party payer is either the government insurance program Medicaid or a managed care organization. Medicaid only reimburses services performed by those they consider to be "providers." A provider is generally defined as a health care worker with a medical or related degree (such as a nurse practitioner), national certification, and a provider number (obtained from the state). The likelihood of reimbursement is largely controlled through the state. Managed care organizations, such as HMOs, use similar criteria. State Medicaid agencies are billed using an HFCA 1500 form incorporating information such as the International Classification of Diseases ICD-9 code, the Current Procedural Terminology (CPT) code, charges, and patient and provider information. Typically a LC may include HCPCS codes for breast pumps.

Private practice issues

The majority of lactation consultants in private practice must be aware of local restrictions on operating a home business or advertising on the premises. Business promotion is often an issue as most lactation consultants have no prior business experience. Another concern is whether or not to incorporate or to form a partnership. Incorporation involves monetary outlay and regulation at the state and federal level, but it can offer tax benefits and the ability to sell or transfer the business. The decision to form a partnership is dependent on each individual's style, the meshing of those styles, and clearly stated partnership

- 108 -

goals. Another important area is the setting and collection of service fees. Fees should be set based on comparison to other local professionals, business overhead, and the length of the service. The latter should incorporate additional amounts for travel if services are performed in the patient's home. The client is generally billed directly at the time of service, and she, in turn, should deal directly with any third-party payers. Private practice LCs who rent or sell breast pumps should be conversant about their use.

Breastfeeding Equipment and Technology

Optimal breast milk expression

Optimal breast milk expression occurs with favorable conditions for stimulation of the milk-ejection reflex in which oxytocin is secreted. First of all, the woman should be relaxed at the time of expression. The milk-ejection reflex should be elicited a minute or two before pumping is begun by using techniques such as massaging the breast with a warm, hot cloth or taking a hot shower. The milk yield can be increased by external compression to each quadrant of the breast during the pumping which creates positive pressure inside the breast and a gradient for milk flow. This massaging is not point compression, which may induce injury to the breast. The vacuum should only be used for short periods to maintain flow, and inserts can be used to get the best fit between the pump and the breast. Once the milk ceases flowing, the breast pump should be removed to avoid tissue damage.

Breast pumping

The user should be familiar with directions for use and cleaning of the breast pump before expression begins. They should wash their hands before beginning. If possible, pumping should be started within 6 hours of delivery. If pumping is being utilized because the infant is premature or ill, the mother should pump at least 8-10 times a day for the first 2 weeks. Expression is usually greatest in the morning, and it generally decreases as the day proceeds. Occasional expression can be down at any time relative to feedings. The pumping time depends to a large extent on the type of pump, with manual pumps requiring 10-15 minutes and electric pumps (usually rented) finished by 15 minutes. There are also battery pumps, which are sometimes used to double pump in a timeframe of 7-15 minutes.

Breast pump types
There are basically 4 types of breast pumps: cylinder, battery-operated, semiautomatic and automatic electric pumps. The concerns for cylinder type pumps are proper use of O rings to maintain suction, cleaning, shape preservation of the gasket or seal, and possible accommodations during the pumping (shortening of pump stroke and/or emptying of the outer cylinder). Battery-operated pumps should be used with alkaline batteries that are changed as soon as the number of cycles per minute diminishes. Recommendations for their use include frequent interruption of the vacuum to prevent nipple pain and injury, choice of a reliable pump (many break down within a few months), and selection of a pump in which the vacuum can be controlled. The breast should be massaged by quadrants during the expression. Semiautomatic pumps are usually selected because there is some degree of control of the vacuum. If an automatic electric pump is utilized, it is recommended that the lowest possible vacuum pressure be used or variable settings be tried during a session. The mother may wish to double pump.

Hormonal considerations and clinical implications
The hormone prolactin, which stimulates lactation, increases greatly during pregnancy (about 200 ng/ml at full-term) and is maintained at relatively high but decreasing levels during the 6 months after delivery if the mother lactates or pumps milk. Lactogenesis II, the onset of milk production during the first few days postpartum, is not dependent on infant

suckling or mechanical milk removal, but galactopoiesis or continued milk production will not occur without one of these methods of removal and stimulation. The mother's breast will become engorged if removal does not occur. Later milk supply is upheld only if there is initiation of early breastfeeding (or pumping), subsequent regulation according to the infant's needs, and a maintenance period of exclusive breastfeeding. Oxytocin, which promotes the milk-ejection reflex through its effects on the myoepithelial cells, is also important. Oxytocin is released in bursts increasing intraductal mammary pressure during suckling or other removal techniques.

Mechanical breast pumps

Mechanical breast pumps work by reducing the opposition to milk outflow from the alveoli thus permitting intramammary pressure from the milk-ejection reflex to push the milk out. The pumps usually have 4 phases: (1) a brief period of increasing suction or negative pressure, (2) a period of decreasing suction, (3) a resting phase, and (4) minimal positive pressure at the end of each cycle. Since suckling infants use suction (half of cycle) and compression (about a quarter into the cycle) during the suckling cycle, milk volumes using mechanical pumps can be increased using similarly timed compression. Examples of mechanical pumps that utilize compressive components are the Whittlestone Breast Expresser and the Whisper Wear breast pump.

Manual breast pumps

Manual breast pumps come in three basic forms: rubber bulb models, squeeze-handle types, and cylinder pumps. Rubber bulb models are increasingly less available and not particularly recommended. A rubber bulb is connected either directly or via tubing to a collection container, and the bulb is squeezed and let go to create a vacuum. They can be problematic due to contamination from backflow and vacuum control difficulty, which causes pain. Squeeze-handle models, such as the Avent Isis and Ameda One-Hand pumps, substitute a handle that produces suction; they are really only appropriate for sporadic pumping. The most common manual pumps are of the cylinder type with two cylinders, an inner one with a flange that is positioned against the breast and an outer one that is drawn away from the body to create a vacuum and fill with milk. There is a gasket between the two cylinders, which creates a seal. Some models have silicone or plastic inserts or liners for fitting. Examples of cylindrical pumps include Evenflo Manual and Ameda Cylinder Hand pumps.

Battery-operated breast pumps

Battery-operated pumps cycle between vacuum suction and release phases, which are either preset or controlled by the mother. They are operated with alkaline batteries (occasionally rechargeable ones) and sometimes have AC adapters to lessen battery use. These are good options for working mothers since they generally do not weigh much and can be controlled with one hand. One major downside is that they usually require frequent battery replacement. Examples include Evenflo Personal Comfort and Lumiscope Gentle Expressions pumps. There is one uniquely designed battery-operated pump, the Whisper Wear pump, which is held in place underneath the bra, works hands-free, and automatically cycles up to 70 times a minute.

Electric breast pumps

There are 3 categories of available electric breast pumps. The first consists of small, semiautomatic pumps, such as the Gerber or Nurture III, which maintain a constant negative pressure. The pumping action is controlled by the mother who uses her finger to alternate between covering and uncovering a hole in the base. Completely automatic electric pumps can be subdivided into 2 other categories, those for personal use and larger ones that are primarily used in institutions like hospitals. Almost all of the automatic pumps cycle pressure. The most commonly used predetermined, pulsed suction ratio of each cycle is 60% negative pressure with a 40% resting phase. There are variations of the basic configuration; for example, the Medela Symphony has a higher cycle stimulation phase at the beginning. Electric pumps generate more negative pressure as the bottle fills up with milk unless there is some sort of compensation mechanism, such as frequent emptying, to maintain constant air volume. An institutionally-used electric pump with a different mode is the Whittlestone Breast Expresser, which has a constant vacuum and compressive phase.

Simultaneous vs. sequential pumping of both breasts

Automatic electric and some battery-operated pumps permit simultaneous pumping of both breasts. Most studies have demonstrated the superiority of simultaneous, double pumping, which mirrors breastfeeding twins, over sequential pumping. Milk yield is basically equivalent but with double pumping, the maximum volumes are achieved much sooner and the total number of hours per week spent pumping are significantly reduced. Some studies indicate that simultaneous pumping may increase prolactin levels, increase milk weight, and/or augment the milk fat concentration.

Pressure generated, hormonal responses, and mechanical issues

The negative pressure created when an infant breastfeeds is slightly lower than all other means of removal except for hand expression, which does not generate negative pressure. Pumps can be controlled over a wide range, however. A baby also creates positive pressure, primarily with their jaw and to a lesser extent with their tongue. A full mother's breast has about 28 mmHg positive pressure, and the milk-ejection reflex generates slightly lower positive pressure. The only pumps that have any positive pressure are electric ones with a compression phase, but hand expression theoretically can have quite a bit of positive pressure. The infant, hand expression, and most pumping techniques have similar maternal prolactin responses. Double pumping as discussed elsewhere can result in higher prolactin levels. A nursing infant can suckle in a range of 36-126 cycles/min and about 0.14 ml upon initiation of feeding which goes down later. These parameters are variable in other means of expression. Pumping generally generates a longer duration of vacuum and fewer cycles.

Flanges

Breast pumps generally have flanges or collars that facilitate breast fit. Flanges are constructed of hard plastic, soft plastic, and silicone. Some pumps have protrusions on the flange that compress the breast or inserts that change the opening diameter. Some pumps include different sized flanges or liners of soft plastic or silicone that are used to manipulate the diameter of the shank and inner opening. Flange options should be selected based on the anatomic configuration and size of the breast, while remembering that nipples swell during pumping. Otherwise damage to the areola may occur. There is some evidence that larger and deeper flanges can better stimulate the areola. Most pumps have a nipple tunnel diameter of 21-40 mm depending on the model and flange option.

Clinical concerns

The biggest clinical concern regarding breast pump use is the risk of bacterial contamination of expressed breast milk. This can occur at a number of levels from cleansing of the nipple or hands to pump cleaning methods. Expressed breast milk is not sterile, and contamination can be minimized. It is recommended that pumps be sterilized between uses, preferably by autoclaving, gas sterilization with ethylene oxide, or high temperature washing or boiling. The collection kit and tubing should be cleaned first, and the exterior of the pump should be washed daily as well. Chemical methods, such as the use of hypochlorite solutions for sterilization, are less desirable because minute quantities of organic material can contaminate the solution. Bacterial counts in milk can also be lowered by early expression initiation, discarding the initial 10 ml of milk (which generally has high counts), and cleansing the nipple and areola with pHisoderm soap prior to pumping. The latter is especially important for expression with non-nursing preterm or high-risk babies because they have immature immune systems.

Storage of expressed breast milk

Storage guidelines for expressed breast milk are based on parameters ensuring acceptable bacterial levels and growth. The acceptable bacterial level for preterm milk is 104 cfu/ml (colony forming units/ml); this allows storage of milk at room temperature (~74-96°F) for approximately 4 hours. Preterm milk may contain protective substances as its storage threshold is greater than that of term milk (3-4 hours). Term infants, however, are more likely to tolerate higher levels of bacteria. Milk stored at a temperature of 59°F can be safely stored for about 24 hours. Storage time increases to 3 days at 39°F (4°C); 2 weeks if frozen in a standard compartmentalized refrigerator; 3-12 months if frozen in a separate freezer at -4°F (-20°C); and longer in a deep freezer -94°F (-70°C).

Breast pump use and reuse

The United States Food and Drug Administration (FDA) monitors the safety and concerns regarding breast pumps and other medical devices. Two databases that report potential problems with medical devices are the Manufacturer and User Facility Device Experience (MAUDE) and Medical Device Reporting Web sites. Both are accessed via www.accessdata.fda.gov/scripts/cdrh/cf docs. Concerns regarding breast pumps should be reported to the FDA at www.fda.gov or via their adverse event reporting program called MedWatch (www.fda.gov/medwatch). The FDA asserts that breast pumps that are not properly sterilized should not be sold or used by another individual. The FDA approves the following breast pumps for use by multiple users: Hollister models (Elite, Lact-e, SMB) and Medela breast pumps (Classic, Lactina). Many models are specifically designed for single users.

Common problems

There are four frequently encountered breast pumping problems. The first is sore nipples, which can be minimized with proper vacuum control. Mothers should use the lowest possible vacuum, delay vacuum until release has begun, and frequently interrupt the vacuum. The mother can also switch sides, use short pumping periods, or find a better fitting flange to minimize sore nipples. The next two problems are interrelated: obtaining small amounts of milk per session and a delayed or irregular milk-ejection reflex. Lack of a milk-ejection reflex is the major reason causing only small amounts of milk collection. These issues may be alleviated by pumping in the morning or between feedings, using a nasal spray containing oxytocin, and pumping under relaxing circumstances. The other frequently encountered problem is a diminishing milk supply over the course of long-standing pumping. Drugs that can enhance milk production in these cases include metaclopromide, domperidone, and human growth hormone; acupuncture has also proven effective for some.

Nipple shields

Nipple shields have been used in various forms for about 400 years. Modern versions are very thin, flexible shields made of latex or silicone resembling a nipple shape with the firmest part being the nipple. Other variations, such as rubber shields or standard bottle nipples (alone or attached to a glass or plastic base), are not recommended. Nipple shields can provide the infant with oral stimulation and a stable, protruding nipple shape. Milk can be extracted by expression without much suction or negative pressure, the milk flow rate may be increased, and the shield helps the baby to learn to feed at the breast. Shields do not correct problems or repair injured nipples. They have a number of disadvantages, in particular insufficient milk volume due to the introduction of a barrier, which somewhat inhibits milk transfer. Nipple shields can also introduce destructive infant feeding patterns, such as shield addiction and later chewing instead of suckling of the breast. If they are not put on properly, the mother can have external or internal breast trauma.

The most common indications for nipple shield use are latch difficulties, oral cavity issues, or upper airway problems in the infant. Another situation is as a last resort for a mother with damaged nipples. There are a number of underlying reasons that cause failure to latch. The child may have problems such as an oral aversion, abnormal tone, or a weak or erratic suckle. The mother may be heavily medicated or have nipple abnormalities. Infant oral cavity problems can include

cleft or other palate issues, a lack of fat pads, inadequate tongue grooving, or a recessed jaw. Upper airway disorders that call for nipple shield use are abnormal softening of tissues in the infant's trachea or larynx (tracheomalacia and laryngomalacia, respectively).

Shields are applied by turning them nearly inside out and wetting the edges to help them to stick to the breast. Some experts suggest encouraging the infant by either trickling expressed milk along the shield, hand expressing small amounts of milk from the teat, and/or breast massage. A shield's teat height should be shorter than the distance between the child's palate juncture and their lip closure so that they do not close their mouth on the shaft. The child should be suckling on the breast, not the tip of the artificial teat. If supplementation is intended, tubing is run either inside or outside the shield. Precautions against contamination include thorough soap washing and rinsing after use or boiling if the mother has yeast on her areola. The infant's weight should be periodically checked to make sure they are getting enough milk and gaining weight. The child can be weaned from nipple shield use by simply removing the shield during feeding or gradually trying to feed without it.

Responsibilities of lactation consultant
Any encounter involving the use or potential use of a nipple shield should be recorded and communicated to the primary health care provider. It is preferable to also obtain written informed consent. Recommendation of nipple shield use can have legal repercussions. The consultant should understand the proper use of and risks involved with nipple shields and be able to adequately instruct the mother. Shield use should not be suggested unless there is a true indication, as discussed previously. Nipple shields are not

appropriate as substitutes for trained care or as quick fixes to initiate breastfeeding. Outside the hospital setting, a referral to a lactation consultant or nurse practitioner is needed when shields are utilized.

Breast shells

Modern breast shells are two-piece plastic contrivances consisting of a base applied over the nipple and areola, and a dome (usually with ventilation holes) placed over that base. Their main use is the eversion or turning outward of retracted or flat nipples. The woman can use the shells during the day before her child is born, after delivery, between feedings, to release engorgement, or in any case where nipple correction is needed. Breast shell use is rarely encouraged by professionals because most shells hold in moisture and heat thereby encouraging soreness and skin damage.

Feeding-tube devices

A feeding-tube device is an apparatus consisting of a container holding breast milk connected to thin tubing, which is attached to the mother's nipple and secured along the areola. These devices are used to temporarily supplement breastfeeding until the infant is adequately established at the breast. Flow is controlled by the child. Feeding-tube devices are indicated if the child exhibits suckling issues or illness. Maternal causes for feeding-tube device use include relactation, induced lactation, inadequate functional breast tissue, nipple trauma, breast reduction surgery, or other illness or surgery. Some of the better known commercially available feeding tube devices are the Lact-Aid and Supplemental Nutrition System (SNS) from Medela. Noncommercial setups can be made from gavage tubing, butterfly needle tubing, or even cups and droppers.

Considerations before recommending use

A baby should theoretically be capable of the latch-on response and some manner of suckling. If they are not, tube feeding is sometimes started by finger use, but that mode tends to encourage wrong suckling patterns. Frequent monitoring by the lactation consultant or other professional is required to guarantee adequate intake and infant weight gain. Weaning needs to be initiated as soon as appropriate because either party may become addicted to feeding-tube use. Thinner tubes can clog if formulas that are not well mixed are used instead of breast milk. The mother must clutch or hold the baby in a manner where she can control the baby's head during tube feedings.

Lact-Aid Nursing Trainer System

The Lact-Aid Nursing Trainer System is a feeding-tube device consisting of a pre-sterilized Lact-Aid bag, an extension tube, a clamp ring, and a body portion with a permanently connected nursing tube. The bag, which sits on a hanger, is filled with breast milk or other supplementation with a funnel. The bag is attached to the extension tube, which is fed through the clamp ring into the body of the Trainer System ending in the flexible nursing tube, and the whole apparatus is attached either to the mother's nursing bra or a neck cord. The infant receives nourishment by suckling both the tip of the nursing tube and the mother's nipple. The baby is prevented from swallowing air by the configuration, particularly the extension tube into the bag.

Storage of human milk

The Academy of Breastfeeding Medicine (ABM) recommends storage in hard-sided containers made of glass or hard plastic for long-term storage and sanctions special plastic bags for short-term use. Their general considerations address cleanliness (hand washing, sterilizing

- 115 -

equipment), small aliquots (2 oz. or smaller), combining chilled expressions, leaving room in the container, and the like. They allow room temperature storage for up to 8 hours and longer with decreasing temperatures. The ABM says the infant can drink the milk cool, at room temperature, or warmed. It can be thawed and then stored in the refrigerator for up to 24 hours. Breast milk is not homogenized and will separate during storage (cream at the top) so the container needs to be swirled before use. Thawed breast milk should not be refrozen. The oldest milk should be used first, and fresh milk is preferable.

Techniques

Early and frequent breastfeeding

Early breastfeeding within the first hour of delivery benefit's the mother in a number of ways. The infant's suckling helps to encourage uterine contractions, the expulsion of the placenta, and modulates the mother's blood loss. Early removal of milk through nursing diminishes maternal breast engorgement and stimulates breast milk synthesis. Lactation is hastened, greater milk production is promoted, and the mother will probably breastfeed longer. Early nursing also has benefits for the infant. A neonate has a powerful suckling reflex to satiate, and the mode offered early (in this case the breast) establishes later behavior. The early colostrum provides needed immunological factors. It provokes peristalsis in the newborn's digestive tract; this is important for the removal of hemoglobin byproducts and reduces the risk of jaundice. Early nursing also improves bonding and attachment between mother and child.

Counseling a new mother

The lactation consultant's primary role in assisting the new mother is to teach the new skill of nursing. The consultant should wash her hands meticulously and make sure she and the mother have privacy. She assists the mother with finding a comfortable position in which to breastfeed. Usually the mother sits in a chair or a raised back bed propped up with pillows. Pillows are also used as needed for additional support. The consultant should be kneeling or seated in order to assist the mother at eye level. Next she aids the woman with positioning the newborn's head in the mother's arms and facing her in order to establish eye contact. The mother should be instructed to hold the nursing breast with the opposite hand behind the areola in a C-hold and direct the breast so the infant can latch-on. Once the mother directs her breast to the baby, she should brush her nipple gently against the child's lips to stimulate mouth opening and the rooting reflex. The consultant can actually help the mother in this instance to quickly bring the baby to the breast precisely when she/he opens the mouth widely. The child's nose should not be in contact with the breast to facilitate breathing.

After the mother has been helped to achieve latch-on, the lactation consultant should then advise the mother that nursing duration and frequency should accommodate the child's desires at these initial feedings. The mother should be taught how to identify the infant's hunger cues. Early hunger cues include squirming, moving arms and legs, rooting, and putting their fingers to the mouth. Later the infant may fuss or appear restless and utter squeaky noises or cry sporadically. Once an infant issues a full cry or turns red, they are in the late stages of hunger and must be consoled before they can latch-on effectively. The mother should also be taught how to recognize when the baby is full. The child is usually satiated when she/he stops suckling, falls asleep, or just releases. The consultant should also teach the mother how to break the infant's suction by putting a finger in a corner of the child's mouth.

Infant feeding positions

The 4 main infant feeding positions are:

- Cradle position - This is the traditional, most frequently used position. The infant is held with both arms underneath. The biggest disadvantage is the lack of control of the child's head, which may wobble.

- Cross-cradle hold - Here the mother cradles the baby with the opposite arm and holds the head with that hand while directing with the same side arm. The infant can easily be brought to the breast and there is good head control, but mothers may find this position awkward.
- Football or clutch hold - The baby is cradled similarly to the cross-cradle position but using the arm and hand on the feeding side. The advantages are good head control and the ability to visualize the child's mouth. This position usually must be taught. It is a good choice for low birth weight, premature, or cesarean birth babies.
- Side-lying position - The mother is lying down on her side propped up with pillows. The child lies down on the bed facing the mother, supported by a roll at his/her back. The mother breastfeeds by directing her breast with the opposite hand. The major advantage is minimization of maternal fatigue, but the mother may have trouble seeing well enough to help attachment and worry about smothering.

Newborns who fail to latch-on

Management guidelines for babies failing to latch-on depend the age of the infant. During the first 24 hours after birth, a full-term neonate does not require any supplementation or breast milk because she/he has excess extracellular fluid. Usually interventions include holding the child skin-to-skin and repeated attempts to initiate breastfeeding every 3 hours. If latch-on has not occurred by 18-24 hours, electric pumping (8 times a day) or hand expression is initiated. If latch-on is absent at 24-48 hours postpartum, other interventions may be added, such as feeding with 10-15 cc of expressed breast milk mixed with water, use of alternative feeding methods like finger feeding or spoons, or use of a nipple shield. After 48 hours, previous strategies should be continued and attempts to breastfeed may be done more often, as frequently as every 2 hours. If needed, feedings with expressed breast milk, with or without formula should be larger, about 30-60 cc.

Assessment of nipples and breasts
Some mothers have nipples that are initially too large for the neonate, generally necessitating feeding by spoon or another method until the baby grows. Women with large breasts may have trouble coordinating and positioning during feeding. Securing the baby in such a way as to free up the mother's hands may be helpful. The most common reason mothers have trouble with latching is that their nipples are flat, inverted, or they draw in when the child compresses the breast. These types of problems can be averted through tactics like shaping the breast tissue during latch-on attempts, drawing back the tissue to make the nipples project, pumping the breasts prior to feeding, or using devices such as nipple shields, nipple expanders, or nipple shells between nursing periods. Sometimes the problem is related to engorgement and a little expression with soften up the breast, which encourages a latch.

Possible causes
An infant can have difficulty with latch-on for a number of reasons. Any abnormality in the mouth, such as cleft palate, can impinge the ability to attach. Any situation that makes it difficult for the baby to breathe can prevent feeding. This can be a physical problem like laryngomalacia or tracheomalacia, which respectively impede inspiration and expiration. Likewise, simple nasal

obstruction may affect latch. Nasal stuffiness can be addressed with saline or hydrocortisone drops. Moreover, pressure on the back of the infant's neck causes the baby to worry about nasal obstruction. Breast refusal is often related to birthing pain, trauma, or effects of labor medications. Some neonates have hyper gag reflexes, which may be overcome through practice sucking on the mother's finger. Additionally, the child may position his/her tongue incorrectly. Undesirable stimuli (sight, sound, smell, and others) can cause an aversion to breastfeeding. Regardless of the cause of difficulty, skin-to-skin contact should continue and other means of feeding should be used until the child will breastfeed.

Neonatal feeding patterns

If a neonate awakens and feeds effectively within 3-5 hours of their last meal, the feeding pattern is normal and no intervention is indicated. If they do not fit into this pattern, the infant should be awakened gently, their diaper changed, the baby should be rocked and massaged, and then the breast should be offered. If at that point the child feeds effectively, no further interventions are needed. If they do not breastfeed successfully, then the neonate should be assessed for signs and symptoms of hypoglycemia, sepsis, dehydration, or other issues that might affect feeding. If there are none, then the clinician should wait an hour and then repeat the cycle of waking, diaper changing, massaging, and offering the breast. If, however, the child does show signs of the issues previously mentioned, these findings should be reported to the physician and appropriate supplementation per facility policy should be initiated.

First 5 days after birth and later

During the first five days after birth, a neonate should consume increasing amounts of breast milk. On a per feeding basis, the amounts on days 1, 2, 3, 4, and 5 should be up to 5 cc, 5-15 cc, 15-30 cc, 30-45 cc, and 45-60 cc respectively. On a daily basis, these amounts translate to up to 1 oz, 1-4 oz, 4-8 oz, 8-12 oz, and 12-18 oz. For weeks 1-10, the desired daily milk intake is calculated by multiplying the infant's weight in pounds by 2.5, which represents the preferred daily intake in ounces. Thus a 9 lb infant should consume about 22.5 ounces of milk daily (9 x 2.5). Later, the child requires less milk on a per weight basis.

Problems with feeding near-term neonates

A near-term neonate is a baby born at 34-38 weeks gestation. In most cases, these newborns are treated as full-term infants. However, breastfeeding near-term neonates can be difficult. Their neurological responses and sleep patterns are usually erratic; their cycle of suckling, swallowing, and breathing may not be completely mature; and they often have poor muscle tone. Special interventions, including feeding at longer intervals (every 4 hours), nursing in a position that supports the head, reducing stimulation, maintaining skin-to-skin contact, and keeping the baby warm, may be required. These newborns often cannot get enough milk because they cannot sustain suck/swallow/breathe rhythms. Thus they are often susceptible to hyperbilirubinemia, hypoglycemia, dehydration, and low weight gain. Usually the mother needs to pump milk after nursing and feed it to the child by spoon or cup, both to establish milk production and deliver sufficient calories. Nipple shields are another possible adjunct.

Alternative feeding methods

Both cup-feeding and finger-feeding can be used if the newborn cannot successfully breastfeed. These methods are preferred over bottle-feeding, which can cause rubber nipple confusion. For cup-feeding, the infant is held in an almost upright sitting position and fed with a small cup with a rounded edge. Cup-feeding should not be used for children with a poor gag reflex, neurological problems, or respiratory troubles. Finger feeding can be done by the mother or another individual. Usually a feeding tube device is held close to the end of a larger finger and connected to a syringe or feeding bottle containing expressed breast milk (or sometimes formula). Hands should be clean, and if a glove is used, it should be latex-free. The infant's lips are stroked lightly until the mouth opens; then the person doing the feeding slides in their finger until the tip meets the hard and soft palate juncture. The feeder can sense whether the child is sucking effectively by feeling a pulling along their nail bed, and then milk transfer can be pushed with the syringe. Color, vital signs, and milk transfer amounts should be monitored.

Nipple shield use with newborns

A thin silicone nipple shield applied over the mother's nipple provides a lot of advantages until the infant becomes proficient at breastfeeding. The mother establishes a milk supply by pumping up to 6 times/day after breastfeeding. The shield is used in conjunction with a feeding tube device, which is fed under the shield and attached to a syringe containing the supplemental milk. This technique is useful for infants with weak suckle, difficulty latching-on, or who have become used to bottle-feeding. The infant can receive milk directly from the breast as well as the supplemental milk, which is usually given only as an immediate reward for successful (or attempted) latching-on and suckling. Thus, the child receives additional calories and also learns how to breastfeed.

Hypoglycemia in newborns

Depending on how one defines hypoglycemia in the newborn, a large percentage of neonates could be considered hypoglycemic. A fetus usually receives uninterrupted glucose feeding from the placenta, but after birth, the newborn only gets discontinuous amounts through feeding. Certain classes of neonates have difficulty handling this and need early, frequent feedings to stabilize glucose levels. These can include infants born to mothers with diabetes, low birth weight babies, small-for-gestational-age newborns, postmature neonates, large-for-gestational age infants, and the smaller of twins. Stressful conditions present at or after birth can also induce hypoglycemia including sepsis, asphyxia, and cold stress. If the mother is given hypertonic glucose infusions during labor, neonatal hypoglycemia may be induced.

Various authors have defined neonatal hypoglycemia in terms of serum or plasma glucose levels relative to postnatal age. During the first 24 hours of life, cutoffs for hypoglycemia have been defined as anywhere from <30-40 mg/dL glucose. Levels during the next few days range from <40-45 mg/dL glucose. According to the Academy of Breastfeeding Medicine, term infants do not need to be monitored for glucose levels, and they generally only develop symptoms of hypoglycemia as a result of an underlying illness. Blood glucose levels (obtained through a heel stick) should be monitored in at-risk or symptomatic newborns. Symptoms include trembling, irritability, overblown reflexes, seizures, quick breathing, sluggishness, hypothermia, a poor suck, and/or refusal of breastfeeding. These screening tests should be done within a half-hour of birth for neonates born to mothers with diabetes and within 2 hours for other at-risk infants. Tactics like maintenance of skin-to-skin contact and early breastfeeding can help stabilize blood glucose levels.

Effects of cesarean birth

Nursing rates do not differ significantly in mothers delivering by cesarean birth and those delivering vaginally, but cesarean birth does generally delay lactogenesis and the onset of breastfeeding. This is mainly due to the time required to recover from the surgery and the stress, pain, and risks involved. Lactogenesis and milk transfer cannot be enhanced in the initial postpartum period, and the neonate is often lethargic due to contact with pain medications or anesthesia given during labor. The lactation consultant can assist the mother who has undergone a cesarean surgery in holding her baby and initiating breastfeeding once she is conscious and attentive. Initially the mother can use either the cradle position to hold and feed the baby, or the clutch hold if she is concerned about touching her incision. By 2-3 days after delivery, a side-lying position is often used.

Early postpartum period

Breast engorgement
After giving birth, hormonal shifts induce rapid milk production. This generally causes breast engorgement peaking 3-5 days postpartum. More extreme engorgement can be caused by use of supplements, delayed or limited feedings, removal of the baby from one breast to feed at the other, or breast implants. Maternal fever of unknown etiology is often a sign of engorgement. There are various means of addressing breast engorgement espoused by different experts. Some feel that the only effective means of treatment is use of anti-inflammatory drugs, but other suggested treatments include heat treatments before breastfeeding, cold treatments after breastfeeding, breast massage

followed by milk expression, application of cabbage leaves, ultrasound treatments, and pumping. The mother should attempt to breastfeed frequently to alleviate the pain of engorgement and also use hand expression or electric pumping if necessary.

Breast edema
Breast edema is caused by receipt of excessive amounts of intravenous fluids during childbirth and is characterized by hard breasts and swollen nipples. Thus the newborn cannot latch-on easily. Breast edema can be alleviated through a technique called areolar compression or reverse pressure softening. The technique shifts excess interstitial fluid toward the routes of natural lymphatic drainage, reduces pressure within the milk ducts diminishing latch discomfort for the child, facilitates the ability of the infant to bring the breast into their mouth, and triggers the milk-ejection reflex by stimulating nerves in the nipple and areolar area. Areolar compression is a multi-step process. Initially, pressure is applied with the index finger and thumb to the areolar area until the swelling subsides, and some tissue is softened. Presence of edema is indicated by a finger imprint. This pressure is then applied behind the softened areas while also pressing the chest wall. The goal is to make the areola supple and the nipple pliable enough to accommodate the infant, which can take up to a half hour.

Hand expression

Hand expression is a very effective method of inducing the milk-ejection reflex and compressing the breast for milk removal. The mother is seated with a clean collection cup under her breast. Initially she uses a warm, moist towel to encourage milk flow and gentle breast and nipple massage in a circular motion to induce the milk-ejection reflex. Then she lightly squeezes the breast by pulling her hands forward from the chest toward nipple. The mother then presses into the breast about an inch in back of the nipple using her thumb and forefingers on opposite sides. She alternates pressure and release as needed to obtain the breast milk which drips into the collection cup. In order to express milk from different ducts, she should periodically change her finger positions. If the milk flow subsides, she should begin expression from the alternate breast, possibly returning to the original breast and switching until she is tired or must quit.

Basic feeding technique guidelines

The new mother should be instructed as to basic feeding technique guidelines for the newborn. These guidelines include feeding the infant frequently with at least 8 feedings a day, offering and retaining the child on the first breast until he/she is satiated or requires the other, and watching for hunger cues from the infant in lieu of clock watching. Practices that interfere with effective breastfeeding or encourage nipple confusion should be avoided; these include use of artificial teats or pacifiers and ingestion of formula, water, or glucose solutions. The mother should be taught how to distinguish sufficient milk transfer; these include audible swallowing, independent awakening to feed, and adequate urine (assessed by diaper monitoring) and stool production. Stooling should be at least 4 times a day by day 3, and the stools should be yellow by about day 4-5.

Expected milk intake and associated voids and stools

On day 1 after birth, a typical newborn ingests 30 ml (range 5-100 ml) of colostrum and has one wet diaper and 1 black tarry stooling. Colostrum intake on day 2 is slightly higher (range 10-120 ml), and wet diaper output is 2. Newborns usually drink 200 ml of breast milk on day 3 and have 3 moist diapers and a bit of green stool. By day 4, milk intake increases to 400 ml and the child typically has 4 wet diapers and 4 loose yellow bowel movements. Average milk intake is up to at least 600 ml on day 5, and the baby should have 6 wet diapers. From day 5 to age 6 months, the average milk intake, number of wet diapers, and number of loose yellow stools per day are 750 ml, 6 or more, and 3-5, respectively.

Assessing adequate milk transfer

The first encouraging sign of adequate milk transfer is an alert infant who cues when he needs to feed and appears full afterwards. The mother should be able to hear the baby swallowing. During the first 2 weeks, the minimum daily suckling time should be at least 160-180 minutes. Adequate hydration is indicated by absence of skin tenting after pinching and wet mucous membranes. Hydration can also be assessed by looking at urine output; adequate milk transfer should produce clear urine and 6 or more wet diapers a day within a week after birth. By day 4-5, the newborn should be passing 3-5 (or more) loose, yellow stools daily, suggesting sufficient nutrient intake. For the mother, the main way to assess milk transfer is to look at her nipple; if transfer is adequate, her nipple will be wet and intact without pain. Reporting of any feeding problems suggests possible inadequate milk transfer.

Signals of too little milk removal
If a breastfeeding infant is not removing sufficient amounts of mother's milk, he will demonstrate indications of hunger. These include frequent crying or whining, restlessness, and irritability. The child may suck his fists or blanket, detach from the nipple frequently, fall asleep without releasing the breast, or move his head while feeding. Inordinately long (more than a half hour) or short (less than 5

minutes) nursing on a side can indicate hunger as can enthusiastic taking of pumped milk or formula right after breastfeeding. Infants usually need more milk and frequent feeds than many mothers understand, and late afternoon into early evening is a period when a cluster of feedings may be necessary. In order to maintain an adequate rate of milk synthesis, enough milk (at least ¾ of supply) must be removed at regular intervals (within 4-6 hours) through feeding, pumping, or expression.

Oversupply of milk

A maximum potential supply of milk per lactation cycle is usually established within a few weeks postpartum. There are cases of too much milk production relative to the baby's needs resulting in infant gagging or choking. In these instances, the child's suck/swallow/breathe coordination should be evaluated first; this is often the real source of the problem, and it may resolve once the infant learns the behavior. If there is true oversupply, strategies include offering only one breast at a feeding and expression from the other, taking the infant off briefly during the let-down period before putting him back on the breast, changing feeding positions, and if necessary, using lactation-suppressing medications. Milk oversupply is often caused by taking the baby off one breast too soon or having a poor feeding position. Some infants feed better in a vertical position or if the mother tilts backward to work with gravity. The main reason to momentarily remove the child during let-down is to avoid infant choking on the rapid spray of milk. Milk supply versus infant needs usually equalize around 6 weeks of age.

Nipple pain

New mothers often have transient nipple soreness or pain peaking sometime during the first week postpartum. Protracted, abnormal pain that persists after the first week to 10 days is an indication of an underlying problem. Early nipple and breast pain is usually due to mechanical reasons or physical trauma. The mechanical reasons are generally associated with the infant's oral configuration or suckling pattern, which traumatizes the skin or breast. This trauma can also be caused by poor breastfeeding positioning, rubbing of retracted nipples inside the child's mouth, incorrect breaking of suction by the mother, or milk stoppage and overfull breasts. It can also result from improperly fitted breast shells, nipple shields, or breast pump flanges as well as too much pump pressure for expression. The underlying cause can also be a dermatological situation such as allergies, sensitivity to topical preparations, eczema or psoriasis, infections, particularly *Candida* or other yeast infections, *Staphylococcus* infection (the major source of infectious mastitis), other bacterial colonization (possibly in association with breast abscesses), and herpes simplex virus.

Assessment

If a mother is experiencing nipple pain, there are a number of pertinent observations to make and questions to ask the mother. The most basic observation is the ability to root, which is indicative of readiness to feed and proper nerve response. The infant's mouth should open up during feeding to angle of least 130°. His cheeks should be plump and rounded; if they are puckered, high intra-oral pressure or poor latching exists. The child's tongue should be slightly visible above their lower lip, not retracted. The mother should be aware that her nipple is elongating during feeding. A proper suckling sound should be evident; this is characterized by quiet swallowing every one to three sucks; other noises indicate tongue sucking or an imperfect seal. A secure seal should be created by cupping of the baby's tongue around the nipple, not merely outward flanging of the lips. The suckling pattern generally becomes slower during feeding, but it should be regular. At the end of a normal feed, the mother's nipple should be wet, undamaged, and undistorted.

Distorted nipples after feeding

When a mother's nipple is creased, cracked, red, or otherwise distorted after feeding, it is usually caused by trauma related to a mechanical problem. Often this can be fixed by changing the infant's position during feeding or through therapy to deal with a poor suckling pattern. A common physical problem of the infant that can cause mechanical trauma is ankyloglossia, a so-called tied tongue that has a short, tight frenulum membrane. A surgical procedure called frenotomy or frenuloplasty, cutting of the frenulum, can be done to correct this abnormality. Nipple pain not associated with distortion is almost always linked to infection or some sort of inflammatory disorder.

Treatments

In most cases of cracking, bruising, or other distortion of the nipple and areola, simply washing the area with clean water and saturating the crack with freshly expressed milk is sufficient. Some experts recommend topical antibiotics for infection and topical steroids for inflammation, mainly because *Staphylococcus aureus* infections are often the cause of severe nipple soreness. Breastfeeding should continue unless the pain is quite severe or bleeding or cracking worsens. There is a wide variety of nipple creams and gels available. Most treatments have not been studied well enough to unequivocally recommend their use, but the vast majority of these are relatively cheap and not harmful. Some of the most commonly used types of nipple creams and gels are lanolin-based

or hydrocolloid dressings called hydrogels. Petrolatum-, beeswax-, and glycerin-based products, tea bags, adhesive wound dressings, and food oils have all been used for painful nipples; most of these are drying or have allergenic potential.

Soreness only at latch-on or at the beginning of pumping can be addressed by discontinuing soap or antiseptics for cleansing, use of lanolin or hydrogen, or wearing a 100% cotton bra. If the mother experiences discomfort when the child grasps her breasts or draws in her nipples, she is having trouble with the milk-ejection reflex, which can be stimulated through prior massage and relieved with cold application. Crescent-shaped fissures or blanching suggests that the infant is pinching the nipple or moving up and down; this can generally be addressed by repositioning. Maternal use of breast creams can cause soreness due to allergic reactions; these creams should be discontinued until further evaluation. If soreness occurs because the nipple sticks to the mother's bra or breast pad, then these should be moistened before removal to protect the keratin skin layer. A breast shell may also be useful. The intervention for red nipples depends on the area of discoloration and degree of persistence. A mother with slightly red, chapped nipples just needs reassurance. If the redness extends beyond the nipple/areola area and the mother is in pain throughout feeding, candidiasis is indicated and topical antifungal medications should be applied. If this does not work, referral to another health care provider as well as topical and systemic antibiotics are probably necessary. Persistent, sore nipples that will not heal are usually related to infant issues. If infant clicking sounds or tongue retraction are found, the baby is either sucking his own tongue or has a shallow latch, which can be corrected by positioning the breast deep in the infant's

- 124 -

mouth, bringing their tongue forward, and ensuring outward flanging of the lips. The child may have physical problems that can be corrected, such as ankyloglossia (addressed elsewhere).

Milk stasis

Shortly after giving birth, hormones stimulate lactogenesis and breast milk production resulting in breast engorgement. If milk is not removed through breastfeeding or other means, milk stasis or breast milk retention occurs. The mother with milk stasis feels very painful breast fullness. If the stasis reaches a point where the breast cannot store any more milk, then involution starts and milk synthesis is depressed. The milk must be removed by nursing, hand expression, and/or pumping in order to maintain milk synthesis and prevent complete involution. Otherwise, there is a moment when the process of involution cannot be reversed because the lactocytes are turned off or destroyed. Milk stasis can also cause plugged ducts, breast inflammation, infectious mastitis and abscesses.

Japanese breast massage

The technique of Japanese breast massage is used to improve milk supply and alleviate plugged ducts. First the mother massages the base of her breast. She then holds up the breasts with her thumbs at the armpits and the other fingers propping up the breast from the side. The elbows are shifted back to push the chest forward, and the breasts are pressed toward the center. The rationale is the supposed improvement of milk flow at the base. The next step is to rotate the breast with both hands for 1-2 min. The steps in which the base and center of the breasts are massaged and pressed are repeated. Then the breast is held and squeezed before the initiation of breastfeeding. Another massage

technique suggested by the La Leche League for relaxation or discomfort is to have the mother sit down while the consultant or someone else uses their knuckles to massage from the base of the neck to below the shoulder blades.

Pacifiers

Global initiatives such as the Baby - Friendly Hospital Initiative and most experts disdain use of pacifiers in conjunction with breastfeeding unless used therapeutically. In reality, the majority of breastfeeding mothers utilize pacifiers occasionally, most commonly to defer the time between breastfeeds. The lactation consultant should only encourage pacifier use for reasons that have sound, research-backed therapeutic utility. Therapeutic uses include concurrent usage with tube feeding in preemies, to relax a child who has consumed a large full feed, and to establish different tongue and oral muscle contraction patterns. Routine use of pacifiers is shunned because they can cause a multitude of problems including dental issues, neurological problems, and inability to attach correctly.

Breast refusal or latching problems

Prevention and management
Early problems with infant breast refusal or latch-on can often be prevented through education prior to childbirth. Infants who are put to the breast within an hour of delivery, kept with their mother (if possible with skin-to-skin contact), and handled gently and patiently seldom refuse the breast. If the child cannot latch-on or suck normally, then the causes need to be elucidated. Latching difficulties due to prematurity, illness or facial or oral abnormalities require input from other professionals. If latch-on and sucking are not accomplished within a few days, the primary physician should be consulted. Most other problems can be

- 125 -

addressed by the lactation consultant. For example, if a mother's nipple configuration is the source of the problem, they can use strategies like breast massage, drawing out the nipple with pumping or expanders, or brief use of nipple shields. Babies who are drowsy from labor medications can temporarily be given calories via expressed milk or colostrum preferably while maintaining skin-to-skin contact.

<u>Abrupt refusal after successful breastfeeding</u>

Abrupt breast refusal after previously successful breastfeeding can be due to infant or maternal problems. Infants exhibit this behavior in reaction to injuries, pain, ear infections, teething or other oral problems, other medical issues, or social situations that distress them. After previous effective breastfeeding, maternal issues are usually new-found. For example, the taste of milk can differ if there is a diminishing milk volume or if the mother eats certain foods, takes new drugs, or develops breast cancer. Maternal infectious mastitis, breast abscesses, or pregnancy can cause later breast refusal. During these periods, it is the role of the lactation consultant to figure out a suitable way to still feed the infant (unless they are ready to wean) without resorting to excessive use of pacifiers or bottles. Strategies include feeding expressed milk via spoon or cup, supplementing with soft foods or liquids in the same manner, increasing skin contact, and finding times (such as right before bedtime) when the child is receptive to breastfeeding.

Colic

Infants cry as a late sign of hunger or if they are injured or ill. Colic, on the other hand, is excessive crying and irritability distinguished by a high-pitched scream. It is probably due to spasmodic abdominal cramping as a result of allergic reactions to cow's milk or other foods, gastroesophageal reflux, breastfeeding problems, or exposure to smoke. Up to 6 months of age, management of colic is a multistep process involving purification of the infant's diet (nothing but breast milk) for 2-3 weeks; having the mother keep a diary of her intake for several weeks, monitoring medications taken by both mother and child, as well as noting nursing patterns and infant behavior. The diary is then assessed for emerging patterns and allergy symptoms. If no pattern is identified, referral to an allergist, gastroenterologist, or other expert is appropriate. If a pattern of cow's milk allergy is suggested, the mother should avoid cow's milk and gradually reintroduce cheeses and then other dairy products. Various investigators have found that colic may also be alleviated by certain carrying positions (back, chest or prone), swaddling, or feeding sucrose.

Breastfeeding in multiple birth situations

Full-term twins or triplets should be assessed at the breast individually. If there are no problems, two infants can be fed simultaneous using the football position (both heads toward the center), the cross hold (both heads near the arms), or a mixed position of the two. The mother may require assistance in holding the heads during latch-on. There are special larger pillows designed for simultaneous feeding. If she prefers, the mother can single feed each. Mothers of preterm, ill multiples should begin simultaneous breast pumping until the newborns can breastfeed. The lactation consultant (LC) should elaborate a plan for each multiple's conversion to breastfeeding. There are reports of quadruplets being nursed for at least a year, so with careful planning and charting, most multiples can be breastfed. If caregivers or household workers are employed, it is important that the mother

- 126 -

retain the attachment and feeding roles. The LC should also be attuned to the mother's mood as multiple births create stress, and maternal anxiety disorders are common.

Human milk feeding

Human milk feeding is the provision of expressed human milk in addition to partial breastfeeding. The expressed milk is given at the end of breastfeeding or as a replacement for one or more feedings a day. The practice is primarily used by mothers of multiple infants, especially those with more than 3 babies, or those with infants who have chronic illnesses. Human milk feeding is a good feeding strategy for mothers of multiples because it does not employ other types of supplementation; thus allowing direct breastfeeding later. There are reports of mothers sustaining lactation and human milk feeding for a number of months.

Breastfeeding during pregnancy

Most mothers can successfully breastfeed a child of 6 months or younger while sustaining a subsequent pregnancy. However, the mother may experience hormonally-induced nipple tenderness and breast pain, fatigue, a diminishing milk supply, and uterine contractions during nursing. The taste of her breast milk will probably be altered due to hormonal changes that decrease the lactose content and increase the sodium levels. These and other changes contribute to the observation that many of the nursing children wean before their sibling's birth. In order to maintain both pregnancy and nursing a child, the mother must make sure her diet is nutritious and supplies enough calories; she may require supplemental vitamins.

Public Health

Adolescent mothers

There is no inherent reason why an adolescent mother should not breastfeed. She can produce breast milk similar in composition and volume to an adult. Nevertheless, adolescent mothers tend to breastfeed at a lower rate than adults and for briefer periods. The reasons are primarily psychosocial in nature, such as feelings of failure, lack of privacy, concern about keeping her figure, and isolation. One of the biggest detriments can be the mother's living situation and the way in which her needs are intertwined with those of others. A number of studies have demonstrated that providing education regarding breastfeeding, peer group interventions, support groups, and role modeling can improve the rates of nursing in adolescents. Other evidence indicates that the primary concerns of adolescent mothers are similar to those of older mothers and that her baby's needs are usually her top priority.

Low-income mothers

In industrialized countries, low-income mothers are less likely to breastfeed than more prosperous ones. Breastfeeding rates are improved if the low-income mother is married, has a minimum of a high school education, began prenatal care early, and is either white or Hispanic. Breastfeeding rates in this group have been positively related to factors like partner approval and prior use of breastfeeding by the maternal grandmother. Various studies have shown that low-income mothers are receptive to breastfeeding if given sufficient prenatal and postpartum instruction through multiple classes and/or interaction with a lactation consultant. Adolescent mothers often fall into this low-income group.

Violent situations and childhood sexual abuse of mothers

Literature related to mothers living with domestic violence is scant and equivocal although there is some evidence that breastfeeding rates are low in these situations. The lactation consultant is obligated to contact authorities if she believes domestic violence is occurring. Women who were victims of childhood sexual abuse may have difficulties bringing the child to the breast. They may experience posttraumatic stress disorder because breastfeeding elicits recall of the horrific events. Yet other studies have shown that mothers who were sexually abused might be more likely to breastfeed because they view the practice as part of good parenting. When counseling these women, the lactation consultant should be tactful and respectful when approaching the subject, and she should include suggestions on how to make nursing comfortable along with normal instruction. The LC might suggest milk expression as an alternative to breastfeeding. It is advisable to refer the mother to a mental health provider in order to address her current and/or previous traumatic experiences.

Breastfeeding goals in *Healthy People 2020*

Healthy People 2020 is an updated version of an earlier document (1979) promoting better health for Americans. It was written by the U.S. Department of Health and Human Services (USDHHS). The original document espoused a 75% breastfeeding rate at hospital discharge and 35 % rate at 6 months. The new version of *Healthy People 2020* set higher goals for 2020. Those goals are a 81.9% rate of initiation of breastfeeding in the early postpartum period, a breastfeeding rate of 60.6% at 6 months after delivery, and a nursing rate of 34.1% at infant age of 12 months.

WIC

The WIC program, officially called the Special Supplemental Nutrition Program for Women, Infants, and Children, is a U.S. governmental agency founded in 1972. Its purpose is to supply low-income mothers and their infants with free nutritional counseling and food supplements, including formula. This focus on supplementation inherently seems to discourage breastfeeding. However, the Child Nutrition and WIC Reauthorization Act of 1989, increased funding, promotion, and support for breastfeeding and breastfeeding education. Nevertheless, breastfeeding rates among those receiving WIC aid are still less than in populations not receiving WIC funds.

U.S. policies regarding breastfeeding

The United States Breastfeeding Committee was established in 1998 to increase awareness of the benefits of breastfeeding and make recommendations to increase breastfeeding rates. *The Breastfeeding Promotion Act* was instituted by Congress in 2001, to guard against workplace discrimination of pumping or breastfeeding mothers. Twenty-seven states have legislation that safeguard a woman's entitlement to breastfeed in public or private, and some states relieve nursing women from jury duty. The American Academy of Pediatrics Work Group on Breastfeeding published a policy statement in 1997 promoting breastfeeding, and a number of other relevant professional organizations have issued similar policies since the early 1990s.

International Code of Marketing of Breast-Milk Substitutes

The International Code of Marketing of Breast-Milk Substitutes is a resolution passed in 1981 by the World Health Organization (WHO) (he United States did not vote for this resolution). It is also endorsed by UNICEF, the United Nations International Children's Emergency Fund. The Code was established to provide a model discouraging but not forbidding marketing of manufactured baby milk. The model prohibits advertising, distribution of free samples to mothers and health-care workers, and promotion in health-care facilities of manufactured baby milk. It states artificial feeding methods cannot be idealized in any way on the products, all educational materials must be factual and scientific, and labels should include information about the benefits of breastfeeding and the risks linked to artificial feeding. It prohibits the promotion of inappropriate merchandise, like condensed milk, and sanctions only high-quality, properly stored products. In 1996, WHO voted for 6 more resolutions with further clarifications including mandating that manufacturers of these products underwrite professional education and organizations that monitor compliance.

Innocenti Declaration

The Innocenti Declaration is a 1990 resolution by WHO and UNICEF which reiterates the importance of breastfeeding for the health of both mother and child. The Declaration set 4 goals, which were to be achieved by 1995. The goals were (1) creation of national breastfeeding coordinators and committees, (2) implementation of the WHO International Code of Marketing of Breast-Milk Substitutes (discussed elsewhere), (3) ratification of laws that protect the nursing rights of working women, and (4) practice of the "Ten Steps to Successful Breastfeeding," which had been outlined by WHO in 1989.

Ten Steps to Successful Breastfeeding

The "Ten Steps to Successful Breastfeeding" were developed by the World Health Organization in 1989 as guidelines for facilities that offer maternity services and newborn care. It is incorporated into the Innocenti Declaration and the Baby-Friendly Hospital Initiative. Briefly summarized, the 10 steps are:

- A written, widely distributed breastfeeding policy.
- Training of all health care staff in required skills.
- Giving all pregnant women information about benefits and intricacies of breastfeeding.
- Assist in commencement of breastfeeding within a half hour of birth.
- Demonstrate how to breastfeed and maintain lactation by other means.
- Withhold all other foods from newborns besides breast milk, unless there is a medical need.
- Keep mother and child together round the clock.
- Promote breastfeeding on demand.
- Withhold artificial teats and pacifiers from breastfeeding infants.
- Advance breastfeeding support groups and refer mothers to such upon discharge.

BFHI

The Baby-Friendly Hospital Initiative (BFHI) was instigated by WHO and UNICEF in 1991 as an international effort to promote exclusive breastfeeding. A hospital is considered "baby-friendly" if it follows these practices, which include the "Ten Steps to Successful Breastfeeding." The text of the initiative currently addresses 5 areas: (1) Background and Implementation (on a hospital, national, and global level), (2) Strengthening and Sustaining of the BFHI, (3) Breastfeeding Promotion and Support, including a 20 hour course for maternity staff, (4) Hospital Self-Appraisal and Monitoring tools and guidelines, and (5) External Assessment and Reassessment (only available to assessors). . In the last few years, additional recommendations were added regarding children of HIV-infected mothers (2003) and an expanded view was developed in 2002 as the WHO/UNICEF Global Strategy for Infant and Young Child Feeding. At present, there are more than 20,000 designated BFHI facilities in 152 countries. Compliance is monitored by an external review board.

2002 WHO/UNICEF GSIYCF

The Global Strategy for Infant and Young Child Feeding (GSIYCF) (2002) is an expanded version of the goals of the Baby-Friendly Hospital Initiative (BFHI) put forth by WHO and UNICEF. It reiterates the urgent need for support of good breastfeeding practices and has 9 elements, which are summarized below. Some of the elements are new or have been modified from the original BFHI. The elements include:

- Appointment of national breastfeeding coordinators and committees.
- Adherence to the "Ten Steps to Successful Breastfeeding."
- Promote the International Code of Marketing of Breast-Milk Substitutes.
- Enactment of national legislation protecting working women who breastfeed.
- Development and implementation of a comprehensive feeding policy.
- Take measures to support exclusive breastfeeding until age 6 months and continued nursing for 2 years or more.
- Endorse appropriate

complementary feeding along with continued breastfeeding.

- Supply guidance related to difficult issues, such as parental HIV infection or emergencies.
- Take a forward look in terms of legislation and other measures related to goals of the International Code of Breast-Milk Substitutes and the World Health Assembly.

HIV and Infant Feeding - Framework for Priority Action

The "HIV and Infant Feeding - Framework for Priority Action" document was developed in 2003 by several United Nations agencies. It recommends 5 actions needed to guarantee successful counseling of the HIV-positive mother in terms of infant feeding. Briefly summarized, they direct:

- Development or revision of national infant and young child feeding policies to include HIV.
- Execution and enforcement of the International Code of Marketing of Breast-Milk Substitutes and World Health Assembly Resolutions.
- Promotion and support of appropriate infant and young child feeding practice and encouragement of practices that prevent HIV transmission in the context of Baby-Friendly Hospital Initiative practices. Recommends BFHI or similar breastfeeding training prior to training specifically related to advising the HIV-positive mother.
- Level of support to HIV-positive women should be enough for them to make and carry out appropriate infant feeding decisions.
- Back and publicize research on

HIV and infant feeding.

Specific Chronological Period Issues

Preterm infants

Guidelines for collection to feeding of EMM

Expressed mothers' milk (EMM) is temporarily necessary for preterm infants. All collection equipment should be clean and sterilized daily by boiling in water 15-20 minutes. Only glass or hard plastic containers should be used. The mother should thoroughly wash her hands and wipe the nipple area with water before expression. Collection containers should be well labeled with date, time, infant name, and medical record number. Milk to be used within an hour need not be refrigerated (preferred). If necessary EMM should be refrigerated or frozen to ensure safety of the milk at the time of intended use; refrigeration is appropriate for feedings within 24-48 hours. Milk should be transported on ice in a cooler. Frozen milk should be thawed for 20 minutes in a warm water bath and never refrozen. It is essential to have a designated space in the NICU for milk preparation, gloves should be worn by personnel, and the counter should be wiped after each preparation. Fortifiers are added per doctor's orders, mixed completely without disrupting milk fat membrane integrity, and used within 24 hours. The EMM should be warmed to room temperature for 30 minutes in an incubator before feeding. Maximum feeding time by slow intermittent bolus should be 4 hours.

Feeding of hindmilk

Hindmilk is the latter milk produced during breastfeeding or in expressed mother' milk (EMM). It is higher in calories and fat content than the earlier foremilk. The hindmilk portion can be separated through fractionation. Theoretically, preferential use of hindmilk in preterm infants should advance faster infant growth, but to date, controlled clinical trials addressing this issue have not been done. The caloric and lipid content of these fractions can be estimated using a creamatocrit. Commercial fortifiers still must be added because they contain other necessary supplementation, primarily minerals. Another consideration is that lipophilic medications taken by the mother can pass readily into the fat-rich hindmilk.

Suckling emptied breasts

Having a small or premature infant suckle the mother's emptied breast is a form of nonnutritive suckling that theoretically benefits both mother and infant. The mother gets instant gratification from the child's behaviors and may increase her milk yield. The baby gets the oral stimulation they lack due to tube feedings. The mother expresses her milk and then the infant is placed at the breast using a football or cross-chest position. If Neonatal Continuous Positive Airway tubes are attached, they should be positioned across the mother's lap, extending upward. The goal is merely interaction, not effective suckling, and infant licking and sucking on the nipple tip is appropriate.

Transition from tube feeding to breastfeeding

A natural progression from tube feeding to breastfeeding in preterm infants begins with small amounts of low-flow milk after incomplete breast expression. Often the child has done some nonnutritive suckling at the emptied breast previously. As the baby matures, the mother feeds only later milk where she can control the flow and eventually, when the child can synchronize suckling and breathing, prior expression is unnecessary. Positioning of the premature infant during this process is important because he has weak neck musculature and a heavy head; in order to prevent movements that shut down the child's airway, the head should be supported with a football or cross-lap hold. Since these babies have deficient suction pressures, the infant is actually positioned and held on the nipple.

PIBBS

The Preterm Infant Breastfeeding Behavior Scale (PIBBS) is a tool for a mother of a premature infant that trains her to objectively look at her infant's behavior at the breast. The tool measures factors like rooting, areolar grasp, period of latch-on, sucking, the longest sucking duration, and swallowing. A PIBBS score can range from 1-20. When mothers utilize this scale, studies have shown higher rates of exclusive breastfeeding upon discharge for premature infants born as early as 31 weeks. This type of assessment, or a similar checklist, should be included in medical records for review by other members of the health care team.

Assessment and facilitation of milk transfer: The infant is test weighed before and after breastfeeding. An approximation of milk transfer is 1 gram of weight gain per 1 milliliter of milk consumed. Test weighing should be done when there is apparent milk transfer or if the mother and infant are being discharged. The latter is important because the infant's inadequacies related to suckling can be overcome with an adequate milk supply. If milk transfer is low nearing discharge, it can be increased with maternal use of metoclopramide or domperidone. The mother should also pump milk after breastfeeding sessions for stimulation of milk flow. Silicone nipple shields placed over the mother's nipple during feeding facilitate milk transfer as well. The rigidity of the shields enables the infant to feed using positive compression in lieu of inadequate negative suction pressure. The mother

usually needs to use the nipple shield for 2-3 weeks (including after discharge) until the child's age is equivalent to a term birth. Other strategies are use of cup- or finger-feeding or supplemental nursers.

Discharge planning

The neonatal physician or nurse practitioner usually stipulates a minimum daily milk intake volume for the infant. The child can feed on demand but certain minimal amounts of milk must be consumed within a certain time period, typically 6-8 hours. There are battery-operated scales that can be rented in order to test weigh at home, or the primary health care provider can perform frequent weigh-ins. Discharge planning in the United States differs from that in European in that release usually occurs before the child's full-term birth date, and therefore, many preterm infants are not effectively breastfeeding when discharged. Preterm infants do not commonly consume enough milk for weeks after leaving the hospital and frequent weighing to assess growth and milk transfer is essential. Other methods of milk transfer besides exclusive breastfeeding may be necessary.

Addressing breastfeeding issues

Prenatal period

The primary issues to address during the prenatal period are endorsement of breastfeeding, examination of family perceptions regarding the process, and dissemination of accurate information. The health care provider should obtain a history including previous medical or surgical treatment of the breast as well as family and personal history of breastfeeding. A prenatal breast exam should be performed. The prospective mother should be provided with educational materials and referred to breastfeeding support groups and classes. The relevant issues should be reiterated just after delivery. Any nipple preparation techniques that might induce premature labor should be avoided.

First few days of birth
For the newborn, the main issues for the lactation consultant or health provider are evaluation of the delivery and current needs and education of the mother and family. The weight and gestational age should be recorded. This should include weight loss after birth (3-4 days), which is typically around 8% of birth weight. The history should include a description of the first and subsequent feedings, whether any supplements are being given, the mother's medical state, and whether the baby is voiding (wet diapers) and stooling. A newborn exam should be done including assessments of oral/motor responses, hydration state, and the child's behavioral pattern. The mother should undergo a breast exam. The LC should intervene for problems such as incorrect latch-on or feeding position and low milk supply. Primary issues at 48-72 hours post-delivery are adequacy of the milk supply, infant hydration, and maternal nutrition. Many of the same history and physical assessments should be repeated. Emphasis should be placed on correct breastfeeding or other means of producing milk.

1-3 months of age
By the time the infant is 1 month old, the lactation consultant or health care provider's main goals should be to support the mother and to ensure that milk supply and intake are adequate. At this point, the patient's history should include the infant's feeding pattern, use of supplements, ability to cue, the daily number of wet diapers and stools, the mother's assessment of her milk supply, and other perceptions. The physical assessment should document weight change since birth, observed breastfeeding, and breast and newborn examinations should be done. The health care provider should discuss issues, such as nocturnal feedings, commitment to 6 months of exclusive breastfeeding, elimination patterns, and others, with the mother. The consultant should address issues such as latch-on and feeding position, low milk supply, and supplementation if needed (weight gain <140-196 g/wk or lack of return to birth weight).. The child should be taking 8-12 feeds/day, on cue. At 2 months, many of the same issues should be readdressed. In addition, teething may need to be discussed, and Vitamin D supplementation (100 U/day) may be indicated.

4-6 months of age
When the infant is approximately 4 months of age, the main issues to address are the sustainability of exclusive breastfeeding and its duration. Again a history of feeding pattern, supplementation, and feeding on cue is essential. The issue of working while breastfeeding is relevant at this time. Upon physical exam, the infant should still be gaining 140-196 g/wk, and he/she should be teething. Developmental indicators of readiness for solid foods may be assessed. The child should be feeding 6-12 times/day. This is the time to reiterate the importance of exclusive breastfeeding until age 6 months, possibly in conjunction with supplemental fluids given by cup. Age 6 months is the suggested cutoff for exclusive breastfeeding and time to introduce solid foods. Weekly weight gain should be less at this point, approximately 84-140 g/wk. Some new issues to address are dental hygiene, nursing in public, pressures toward weaning, and iron supplementation for exclusively breastfed infants.

After 6 months of age
The infant's weekly weight gain should drop to about 34-140 g/wk at age 9 months. At this time, breastfeeding

continuance should still be encouraged and the pressure to wean should be discussed. Iron-containing foods should be included in the infant's diet. Starting at 9 months, periodic measurements of hemoglobin (Hgb) or a hematocrit (Hct) might be indicated. From age 9-15 months, the lower limit of Hgb should be 11.3, with a mean of 12.3, and the Hct lower limit is 33.0, with a mean of 35.9. The mother ought to be advised that breastfeeding patterns are variable at this point. At 15 months, it is appropriate to discuss gradual weaning.

Academy of Breastfeeding Medicine protocols

The Academy of Breastfeeding Medicine has developed 12 protocols or plans that can be followed when treating neonates and/or their mothers. Each provides background on the specific topic, recommendations for management, and references. Sometimes risk/assessment parameters, justification for procedures, or prevention techniques are included. The 12 protocols are:

- Guidelines for glucose monitoring and treatment of hypoglycemia in breastfed neonates.
- Guidelines for hospital discharge of the breastfeeding term newborn and mother: "Going home protocol."
- Hospital guidelines for the use of supplementary feedings in the healthy-term, breastfed neonate.
- Mastitis.
- Peripartum breastfeeding management for the healthy mother and infant at term.
- Guideline on co-sleeping and breastfeeding.
- Model breastfeeding policy.
- Human milk storage information for home use in healthy full-term infants.
- Use of galactagogues in initiating or augmenting maternal milk supply.
- Breastfeeding the near-term infant (35-37 weeks gestation).
- Guidelines for the evaluation and management of neonatal ankyloglossia and its complications in the breastfeeding dyad.
- Transitioning the breastfeeding/breast-milk fed premature infant from the neonatal intensive care unit to home

Practice Test

Practice Questions

1. Mammary glands develop in the fetus, beginning with the mammary streak, which evolves into the mammary line or ridge. Where does the mammary line begin and end?
    a. Mammary lines begin below the breast and extend into the axillae
    b. Mammary lines begin in the groin and extend through the axillae into the inner upper arm
    c. Mammary lines begin below the umbilicus and extend to the upper outer breast area
    d. Mammary lines begin at the nipples and extend to the tail of Spence

2. What is a physical change associated with phase 1 of breast development, which occurs at puberty?
    a. Elevation of the nipple
    b. Visible glandular tissue in the subareolar region
    c. Wider and more pigmented areola
    d. Nipple and areola project distinctly from the breast

3. What are the two main arteries that supply blood to the breast?
    a. Lateral thoracic
    b. Internal mammary
    c. Subclavian artery
    d. A and B
    e. B and C

4. The lymphatic system in the breast drains predominantly into the axillary lymph nodes. Which of the following nodes are additional receptacles for lymphatic drainage from the breast?
    a. Parasternal and liver nodes
    b. Intermammary, intra-abdominal, and subclavicular nodes
    c. Cervical and inguinal nodes
    d. A and B
    e. B and C

5. What structures in the nipple and areola cause the nipple to become erect and help in the discharge of milk?
    a. Circular bands of smooth muscle tissue
    b. Increased innervation and blood flow to the nipple and areola
    c. Cooper's ligaments
    d. B and C
    e. A and B

6. A thorough assessment of the breast for a woman who plans to breastfeed includes evaluation of many features. Which of the following could indicate possible problems with breastfeeding?
 a. Asymmetry between breasts, broad spacing between breasts, inverted nipples, scarring, elasticity of skin
 b. Hypoplasia (lack of breast tissue), hyperplasia, thickening in areas of the breast (may indicate tumors)
 c. Teardrop shape of breast
 d. A and C
 e. A and B

7. There are three basic functional reactions of the nipple. Which of the following are included as classifications of nipple function?
 a. Pretraction, movement of the nipple forward
 b. Retraction, movement of the nipple inward
 c. Inversion, nipple is pulled into the areola
 d. B and C
 e. A and B

8. When does stage 1 lactogenesis begin and end?
 a. Second trimester until day one or two postpartum
 b. Third trimester until day two or three postpartum
 c. First trimester until day five or six postpartum
 d. Third trimester until day seven or eight postpartum

9. What are the changes seen in stage 2 lactogenesis?
 a. Increased blood flow
 b. Increased oxygen and glucose absorption
 c. Abundant milk production
 d. Rising pH levels
 e. B, C, and D
 f. A, B, and C

10. The pituitary hormone prolactin stimulates and maintains the production of milk. What hormones directly affect the production of prolactin?
 a. Prolactin-inhibiting factor (PIF) and thyrotropic-releasing hormone (TRH)
 b. Progesterone
 c. Estrogen and dopamine
 d. A and C

11. Oxytocin is a hormone that is present in both males and females. What are the effects of oxytocin on the nursing mother?
 a. Aids in activation of lactation
 b. Produces a soothing effect, lowers blood pressure, and lowers pulse rates
 c. Helps decrease milk production for those who choose not to nurse
 d. A and B

12. The release of milk from the alveoli and minute milk ducts, into the larger lactiferous ducts and sinuses, as a response to suckling, is known as the "let-down reflex" (ejection reflex). This is due to the pituitary glands release of the hormone oxytocin. What effect does oxytocin have on the uterus?
    a. Oxytocin causes the uterus to constrict
    b. Oxytocin causes the uterus to become engorged
    c. Oxytocin has no effect on the uterus
    d. Oxytocin stimulates the engorgement of the endometrium

13. The most important factor in lactation is tactile stimulation. Receptors for what hormones are located in the nipple?
    a. Oxytocin
    b. Prolactin
    c. Estrogen
    d. A and B
    e. A and C

14. Computerized breast measurement (CBM) is a system used to measure milk production without interfering with the infant's breastfeeding schedule. What are the parameters that CBM quantifies?
    a. Variations in breast volume during pregnancy and feeding and volume of milk extracted during feeding
    b. Short-term rate of milk synthesis (S), storage capacity (SC), and degree of fullness (F)
    c. Number of calories provided by the breast milk
    d. A and C
    e. A and B

15. Lactational amenorrhea is the absence of menstruation during lactation. If a woman has intercourse without the use of a contraceptive device during lactational amenorrhea, what is the likelihood of her conceiving?
    a. 20%
    b. 100%
    c. 50%
    d. 0%

16. Your new mother has noticed that her baby has some swelling of her breasts and a few drops of milk like liquid coming from the nipples. How do you explain this phenomena?
    a. She needs to contact her doctor and make sure the newborn does not have excess hormones
    b. Stimulation of the mammary glands of the newborn may result in the secretion of a minute amount of milk from the nipples
    c. The mother should refrain from breastfeeding until the newborn's breast swelling decreases
    d. The baby should be placed on a medication to "dry up" the milk

17. You are discussing contraception with a new mother. She states that she is going back to work when her newborn reaches six weeks of age, and that she will only be able to breastfeed infrequently. She will be supplementing her feedings. Which of the following are factual statements concerning contraceptive use during lactation?

    a. Contraceptive use during lactation does not change the composition of milk, but it can suppress the yield

    b. Most of the time lactating mothers are only started on contraception if they are bleeding, feeding infrequently, using supplementation, and have been tested for pregnancy

    c. High-dosage hormone contraceptives must be used to guarantee contraception

    d. A and B

    e. B and C

18. If the lactating mother becomes pregnant, what is the appropriate response to her inquiry about continuing to breastfeed?

    a. She should stop breastfeeding immediately because the pregnancy hormones will affect the nursing baby

    b. Nursing is contraindicated for pregnant women due to the discomfort

    c. Nursing during pregnancy, known as tandem nursing, does not have a negative effect on the nursing baby, but could stimulate the uterus to contract and cause premature labor

    d. Quick weaning of the baby is preferred

19. Several pharmacologic agents stimulate lactation. Which of the following substances are galactogogues, agents that promote the secretion of milk?

    a. Thyrotropin-releasing hormone

    b. Theophylline (found in coffee and tea)

    c. Depo-Provera

    d. A and B

    e. B and C

20. Relactation is the reintroduction of lactation once it has been discontinued. What are some of the situations that may indicate relactation may be utilized?

    a. Mothers of premature infants who could not be breastfed at birth

    b. Adoption of an infant, after nursing a biological child

    c. Relactation is more likely in women who have undergone complete postpartum breast involution.

    d. A and C

    e. A and B

21. The secretion of prolactin can be depressed by the use of certain medications that increase prolactin-inhibiting factor, or increase its activity. Which of the following pharmacologic agents may be used to inhibit lactation?

    a. L-dopa

    b. Ergot alkaloids

    c. Vitamin B12

    d. A and B

    e. B and C

22. The growth and development of the newborn is directly affected by the mineral content of the milk from the lactating mother. Which of the following statements regarding human milk and cow's milk are true?
    a. Cow's milk contains lower concentrations of sodium, potassium, and chloride
    b. Cow's milk contains nearly three to four times the salt content of human milk
    c. The mean ratio of calcium to phosphorus is higher in human breast milk than in cow's milk
    d. A and C
    e. B and C

23. The Human Milk Banking Association of North America (HMBANA) has established priorities for the distribution of milk from human donors. Which of the following is at the top of the list for receiving this milk?
    a. Full-term newborns weighing less than five pounds
    b. Premature infants who are ill
    c. Full-term infants with heart disease
    d. Healthy premature infants

24. There are several water-soluble vitamins found in human milk. Which of the following are included?
    a. Thiamine, folic acid
    b. Riboflavin, niacin, vitamin B6, B12
    c. Vitamin A, vitamin E
    d. Vitamin C
    e. A and C
    f. A, B, and D

25. The lactating mother should consume a variety of foods to ensure the proper development of her infant. Which of the following statements is incorrect?
    a. Fat consumption should be avoided to prevent atherosclerosis in the mother and infant
    b. Fat consumption is important because it is related to brain and nervous system development
    c. Retinal and neuronal development are dependent upon docosahexanoic acid, which is found in fats
    d. The essential fatty acids, linoleic and linolenic acids, enhance nervous system development by hampering demyelination

26. The stimulation of lactation in a woman who has not recently been pregnant is known as "induced lactation." Which of the following situations are examples of "induced lactation"?
    a. Lactation in a postmenopausal woman who has a child through fertility techniques plus hormone therapy
    b. Adoptive parent who wishes to breastfeed
    c. Lactation in a man
    d. A and C
    e. A and B

27. The capability to swallow develops in week 24 of gestation; consequently, the swallowing reflex is present at birth. Which of the following statements is incorrect regarding newborn suckling?
    a. When the newborn is four days old, sucking and swallowing are perfected
    b. Swallowing occurs between inspiration and expiration
    c. Nearly half of a full feeding is consumed within two minutes
    d. Newborns are mouth breathers, so they stop sucking to take a breath

28. What are some common causes of abnormal suckling patterns?
    a. The use of secobarbital or meperidine during labor
    b. The use of chloroprocaine during labor
    c. C-section delivery
    d. A and B
    e. A and C

29. Human milk has an average caloric content of approximately 65 kcal/dL.
Which of the following statements regarding breastfed infants is correct?
    a. Breastfed infants have a higher percentage of body fat than bottle-fed infants
    b. Mean body weights of breastfed infants are significantly lower than bottle-fed infants
    c. Milk yield from both breasts is nearly equal
    d. Large breasts produce much more milk than small breasts

30. You are consulting with a woman who has delivered a month early. She is concerned that her breast milk will not be sufficiently mature to adequately nourish the baby. Which of the following statements should be included in your advice to this new mother?
    a. The milk from a mother who has a premature infant is higher in calories and nutrients during the first month than the milk of a mother of a full-term infant
    b. Lactose levels are much higher in preterm than in full-term breast milk
    c. Milk from a mother of a preterm infant is higher in calcium, phosphorus, zinc, magnesium and sodium
    d. A and B
    e. A and C

31. The recommended daily allowance (RDA) for a lactating mother is about 500 calories above normal. Since the mother is consuming a high-calorie diet, what prevents excessive weight gain?
    a. Caloric loss when milk is expressed
    b. Basal metabolic rates increase while lactating
    c. Daily exercise program
    d. Lack of sleep

32. The lactating mother should have comprehensive dietary counseling to assure her nutritional health and that of her newborn. Which of the following areas need to be addressed in this session?
   a. Mother's eating patterns, ability to obtain food, actual intake and lifestyle, and her perception of her weight
   b. Intake of calcium-rich foods; food she may exclude (vegetarian diet); and habits such as smoking, drinking, and recreational drug usage
   c. Mother's education level
   d. A and C
   e. A and B

33. Which of the following statements are accurate regarding colostrum, mature human milk, and cow's milk?
   a. Vitamin A levels (for retinal development) are higher in colostrum than in human and cow's milk
   b. Vitamin D levels (for calcium absorption) are low in both human and cow's milk, and higher in colostrum, but supplementation or sunlight exposure is still needed
   c. Human milk has higher levels of vitamin K (for blood clotting) than cow's milk
   d. A and B
   e. B and C

34. Full-term infants usually do not require vitamin or mineral supplementation if their formula is iron fortified. What are the recommendations for breastfed infants?
   a. Breastfed infants should receive 200 IU of vitamin D per day
   b. Breastfed infants do not require an iron supplement
   c. All preterm infants require vitamin/mineral supplementation
   d. A and C

35. Weaning is defined by the World Health Organization (WHO) as the introduction of solid foods, while continuing to breastfeed. Age six months is a good time to introduce solid foods. Which of the following statements support this recommendation?
   a. The infant's iron stores are depleted
   b. The infant's chewing and swallowing reflexes are developed
   c. Rhythmic biting has begun
   d. B and C
   e. A and B

36. The newborn has an immature immune system. What are the immunological advantages of breast milk over cow's milk or formula?
   a. Increases the lymphocyte production of the newborn
   b. Protection against infection, shielding the GI mucous membrane against pathogens
   c. Enhances development of the newborn's immune system
   d. A and B
   e. B and C

37. Human milk affords antibacterial protection through several different means. Which of the following statements is incorrect?
    a. Bifidus factor in human milk sustains the growth of Lactobacillus bifidus
    b. The bacterium Lactobacillus bifidus stimulates antibody production, promotes phagocyte production, and restores the balance of normal flora
    c. Lactoferrin binds to iron to inhibit proliferation of B- and T-lymphocytes
    d. Lactoperoxidase is an enzyme that works in combination with IgA to eradicate Streptococci

38. Mastitis is an infection of the breast that is usually unilateral, characterized by swelling and redness. Which of the following statements are inaccurate regarding mastitis?
    a. Mastitis causes fever of at least 101°F, extreme localized pain, systemic illness, influenza-type symptoms, and cracked and painful nipples
    b. Engorgement or plugged ducts can predispose a woman to mastitis
    c. Antibiotics are unnecessary; mastitis will resolve itself
    d. Emptying the breast is insufficient treatment

39. Diabetic women have a higher incidence of problems with birth. Which of the following occur in infants of diabetic mothers?
    a. Respiratory distress syndrome (RDS)
    b. Hyperglycemia
    c. Inborn malformations
    d. A and C

40. Mothers who smoke heavily frequently have lower birth weight babies. Which of the following statements is inaccurate?
    a. Nicotine suppresses the let-down reflex
    b. Smoking correlates with poor milk volumes
    c. Nicotine and cotinine are found in the smoking mother's milk
    d. Nicotine gum and patches do not transfer nicotine into mother's milk

41. Lactating mothers with staphylococcal mastitis could transfer the infection to their newborn. Which of the following statements is inaccurate regarding staphylococcal infections?
    a. Scalded skin syndrome (SSS) in infants frequently comes from breastfeeding from a mother with staphylococcal mastitis
    b. Methicillin-resistant Staphylococcus aureus (MRSA) is a major concern in nursing newborns
    c. When the lactating mother has a staphylococcal mastitis, breastfeeding should be delayed until a full regimen of antibiotic therapy is completed
    d. Oxacillin and erythromycin are used to treat staphylococcal infections

42. Maternal toxic shock syndrome (TSS) may be fatal if not properly treated. What are the signs and symptoms of TSS?
    a. Fever, rash, and hypotension
    b. Desquamation and multiple organ involvement
    c. Tarry stools, nausea, and vomiting
    d. A and C
    e. A and B

43. Hepatitis C virus (HCV), an RNA-containing flavivirus, may cause an acute infection, chronic hepatitis, cirrhosis, and possibly hepatocellular carcinoma. What are some of the concerns that the clinician should discuss with the new mother with hepatitis C?

a. The possibility of transfer to the infant is low, so the risk is minimal
b. There are no current vaccines or immunoglobulin preparations for HCV
c. If HCV is transferred, the probability of chronicity is high
d. A and C
e. B and C

44. Post mature infants have a unique set of problems, which may lead to difficult suckling. Initially, this infant may need intravenous therapy with a gradual introduction of breastfeeding. What are some of the physical problems the postmature infant may experience?

a. The placenta loses vitality, causing weight loss and decreases in subcutaneous fat and stored glycogen
b. Predisposition to hyperglycemia, hypercalcemia
c. During birth, intrauterine hypoxia or asphyxiation from lack of placental reserve, leading to decreased motility and hormone levels in the intestinal tract
d. A and C
e. B and C

45. The American Academy of Pediatrics has guidelines for the treatment of hyperbilirubinemia. Which of the following statements regarding proper treatment is inaccurate?

a. If the total serum bilirubin (TSB) level is $\geq$ 8 to 10 mg/dL on day two of life, phototherapy is considered
b. If the TSB level is $\geq$ 15 mg/dL on day three, phototherapy is considered
c. For older neonates with TSB levels of $\geq$ 17 to 20 mg/dL, phototherapy is considered
d. If TSB levels continue to rise and phototherapy is ineffective, exchange transfusion is instituted

46. Hyperbilirubinemia in the breastfed infant that is late-onset, occurring at around 5 to 10 days, frequently lasts for more than a month. This type of late-onset jaundice, with a TSB level of > 20 mg/dL, is unrelated to caloric intake or stooling. Which of the following statements is correct?

a. Breastfeeding has no effect on serum bilirubin levels
b. Breastfeeding should be discontinued until tests determine serum bilirubin levels and the effects of breastfeeding
c. Breastfeeding sessions should be cut in half when the TSB level elevates toward 15 mg/dL
d. Breastfeeding should be discontinued permanently

47. Necrotizing enterocolitis (NEC) causes the death of intestinal tissue and frequently occurs in premature infants and newborns that have experienced transient asphyxia, exchange transfusions, or infection with gram-negative bacteria Klebsiella, Escherichia coli, and Bacteroides. Which of the following are symptoms of NEC?
   a. Abdominal distention
   b. Vomiting, diarrhea, and bloody stool
   c. Hematuria
   d. A and B
   e. B and C

48. A mother may need to wean a nursing infant due to an abrupt separation due to "milk fever." What are the symptoms of this condition?
   a. Chills, fever, and dejection
   b. Engorgement and depression
   c. Diarrhea and vomiting
   d. A and C
   e. A and B

49. Which of the following breastfeeding assessment tools and questionnaires are commonly used?
   a. Breastfeeding Attrition Prediction Tool (BAPT)
   b. Breastfeeding Self-Efficacy Scale (BSES)
   c. Maternal Breastfeeding Education Source (MBFES)
   d. A, B, and C
   e. B and C

50. The scope of practice for the International Board Certified Lactation Consultant (ICBLC) includes which of the following tenets?
   a. Provide capable, evidence-based care and maintain records and reports
   b. Uphold professional standards, and use information from each case as examples for others
   c. Promote and support breastfeeding and provide expert services for mother and family
   d A and B
   e. A, B, and C

Answers and Explanations

1. B: The mammary line or ridge begins in the groin area and extends through the axillae into the inner upper arm.

2. A: Elevation of the nipple is the physical change that occurs in phase 1 of breast development. Projection of the nipple and the breast begin in the second phase. Phase 3 includes enlargement and pigmentation of the areola with well-defined glandular tissue. In phase 4, the areola continues to increase in size and coloration, and the nipple and areola clearly project out from the remainder of the breast tissue. In phase 5, the shape of the breast becomes more even.

3. D: The main arteries that supply blood to the breast are the internal mammary artery, which supplies 60% of the blood to the breast, and the lateral thoracic artery. The axillary, intercostal, and subclavian arteries provide additional, but less significant, circulation to the breast.

4. D: The axillary nodes provide the principal drainage for the lymphatic system of the breasts. Additional drainage routes include the parasternal nodes located in the thoracic cavity, the intermammary nodes that lie between the breasts, intra-abdominal, subclavian, and liver nodes. The cervical and inguinal lymph nodes are not connected directly to the breast lymphatic system.

5. E: Rings of smooth muscle are located in the areola and nipple areas of the breast. When this muscle tissue constricts, the nipple becomes erect, and during lactation, this results in the discharge of milk. This region has an abundance of nerve endings, which are in close approximation to the arterioles that supply blood to the nipple and areola. Stimulation of the nipple by temperature change, touch, or sexual contact produces an increase in blood supply, which, in conjunction with the constriction of the smooth muscles, results in nipple erection. Cooper's ligaments provide support for the breast and aid in maintaining the breast's shape.

6. E: Thorough assessment of the breast is necessary for any woman who intends to breastfeed. Obvious asymmetry could indicate inadequate glandular tissue; hypoplasia and hyperplasia, along with broad spacing between the breasts, can affect lactation. Elasticity and turgor of the skin are important aspects of the examination. Any thickening in the breast tissue indicates that further testing for tumors should be done; scars could indicate past surgeries, and a complete history should be taken. A teardrop-shaped breast should not cause any concern.

7. D: There are three basic functional reactions of the nipple: protraction, retraction, and inversion. Protraction describes the movement of the nipple forward, retraction refers to the inward movement, and inversion is the situation in which the nipple remains inside the areola upon observation. In simple inversion, the nipple responds to manual pressure or cold and protracts, and in complete inversion, the nipple is inverted due to scar tissue.

8. B: The first stage of lactogenesis, stage 1, begins during the third trimester of pregnancy and lasts until day two or three of the postpartum period.

9. F: Stage 2 lactogenesis is characterized by an increased flow of blood, citrate levels, plasma a-lactalbumin, increased milk production, free phosphate and calcium concentrations, and a fall in the pH level.

10. D: Prolactin is a pituitary hormone that is influenced by the levels of other substances in the blood. Prolactin-inhibiting factor (PIF) reduces prolactin levels. Thyrotropic-releasing hormone (TRH) has a powerfully stimulating effect on the production of prolactin. Pharmacological agents, such as estrogen, stimulate production, while dopamine inhibits it. Progesterone is a hormone that acts to prepare the uterus for implantation by a fertilized ovum for maintenance of pregnancy, and it aids in mammary gland development.

11. D: Oxytocin, produced by the hypothalamus, triggers lactation in women. It enhances lactation by creating a soothing effect and lowering pulse rates and blood pressure; this creates a more relaxed interface with the nursing newborn.

12. A: Oxytocin causes the uterus to constrict.

13. D: Receptors for both oxytocin and prolactin are located in the nipple.

14. E: Computerized breast measurement (CBM) refers to a technique of measuring milk production without compromising the infant's breastfeeding schedule. CBM measures variations in breast volume during feeding, as well as during pregnancy, and the volume of milk extracted upon feeding. The first parameter is the short-term rate of milk synthesis (S), defined as the increase in breast volume between feedings divided by the time between recorded sessions. Another parameter is storage capacity (SC), described as the difference between maximum and minimum breast volumes during a 24-hour period. Normal values for storage capacity range between 80 and 600 mL. CBM defines the degree of fullness (F), which is the ratio between a specific breast volume and the storage capacity at that time. CBM is more efficient than other methodologies such as weighing the mother and infant, isotope dilution techniques, and use of a breast pump.

15. A: The chance of conception for the woman experiencing lactation amenorrhea is less than 20%.

16. B: Both male and female newborns have the ability to produce small amounts of milk for up to one month. This phenomena is due to the stimulation of their mammary glands by the placental hormones.

17. D: Milk composition is unaffected by the use of contraceptives during lactation; however, the amount of milk produced may be suppressed. The concentration of hormones in the contraceptives should be kept to a minimal dosage. The lactating mother may be given contraceptives if she is experiencing vaginal bleeding, feeding infrequently, using supplemental feedings, and only if she has had pregnancy testing.

18. C: The continuation of nursing for the pregnant lactating mother, known as tandem nursing, is acceptable as long as the mother is receiving an ample amount of calories, so both the fetus and the nursing infant are adequately nourished. The main concern regarding

the continuation of nursing while pregnant is early onset of labor due to uterine contractions caused by nipple stimulation and oxytocin production. If the mother prefers to wean the nursing infant, the process should be done over a long enough period of time to allow for adequate adjustment to the alternate source of nutrition.

19. D: Thyrotropin-releasing hormone (TRH) stimulates the adenohypophyseal lactotrophs, the cells located in the anterior pituitary that produce prolactin. Theophylline can stimulate prolactin secretion and is found in tea and coffee.

20. E: Relactation is often used by mothers of premature or sick infants, who were unable to breastfeed at birth or who developed an allergy or intolerance to breast milk.

21. D: Drugs that decrease prolactin secretion do so by enhancing the activity of or increasing the production of prolactin-inhibiting factor (PIF). L-dopa inhibits prolactin secretion by supplementing the hypothalamic levels of dopamine and catecholamine, which amplifies the activity of PIF. Ergot alkaloids inhibit adenohypophyseal secretion of prolactin and may increase hypothalamic-controlled PIF activity. Vitamin B12 does not inhibit prolactin secretion.

22. E: Cow's milk has between three and four times as much sodium as human milk. The mean ratio of calcium to phosphorus is higher in human breast milk than in cow's milk. Cow's milk contains higher concentrations of sodium, potassium, and chloride.

23. B: The HMBANA, which currently has 10 banks in the U.S., rates the premature infant who is ill as the number-one recipient of human donor milk, followed by healthy preterm infants. Combinations of medical conditions and age decide who takes precedence.

24. F: Water-soluble vitamins that are present in human milk include thiamine, niacin, riboflavin, folic acid, vitamins B6 and B12, and vitamin C.

25. A: Fat consumption directly affects the neural development of the newborn. The brain enlarges threefold during the first 12 months of life; this growth is linked to the integration of long-chain polyunsaturated fatty acids into the phospholipids in the cerebral cortex. Linoleic and linolenic acids enhance the nervous system by obstructing demyelination.

26. E: The stimulation of lactation in a woman who is not recently postpartum is induced lactation. Postmenopausal women who have conceived due to hormone therapy and fertility techniques use induced lactation if they plan to breastfeed. Relactation occurs when a woman gives birth and decides not to breastfeed, or starts breastfeeding, then stops, and later resumes nursing. Inappropriate lactation is lactation that occurs in a man, in a woman who has never had children, or in a woman who has terminated a pregnancy three months or more prior to beginning to lactate.

27. D: Usually by the time the infant is four days old, swallowing and sucking are perfected. The newborn sucks twice as often as he or she swallows, which occurs between expiration and inspiration. Within the first two minutes after beginning to nurse, the infant consumes nearly half of the entire feeding, with most of the feeding completed by four minutes. Most newborns are nose breathers, so breathing during nursing does not pose a problem.

28. E: Abnormal suckling patterns may be caused by the use of meperidine or secobarbital during labor. Infants exposed to these medications frequently have difficulties suckling in their first few days after birth. Chloroprocaine is readily metabolized and has a minimal effect on suckling. Complicated deliveries and C-sections may predispose the infant to breastfeeding difficulties.

29. A: Breastfed and bottle-fed infants' mean body weights are quite similar. Infants who breastfeed expend fewer calories and have a higher percentage of body fat than bottle-fed infants. Women with small breasts produce as much milk as women with large breasts, but larger breasted women have more storage capacity, allowing for more flexibility in their feeding patterns. The milk yield varies between breasts, with the right breast generally producing more than the left.

30.E: Mothers of preterm infants produce milk during the first month after delivery that is higher in concentrations of kilocalories, lipids, protein, fatty acids, nitrogen, some micronutrients, immunoglobulins, immune cells, and anti-inflammatory factors than the milk produced by mothers of full-term infants. Greater levels of calcium, phosphorus, zinc, magnesium, and sodium are found in preterm milk.

31. B: Basal metabolic rates escalate during lactation and prevent the mother from excessive weight gain from the increased caloric intake. The lactating mother should avoid extreme diet practices that can have negative effects on the nursing infant, through the release of fat-soluble toxic materials into the milk. Generally, a diet of 1500 calories a day is sufficient. Moderate exercise accompanied by a diet of 2200 calories per day, and a reduction in dietary fat content to a maximum of 25%, may help with weight loss. Sleep loss may have an effect on the general well-being of the new mother, but the main deterrent for excessive weight gain is the increased basal metabolic rate.

32. E: It is important to discuss the mother's usual eating patterns, her ability to obtain food, and her lifestyle as it influences her nutritional status. The mother's perception of her weight is significant. The content of her diet, including calcium-rich foods, fruits and vegetables, foods she may exclude—including vegetarian diets, and habits such as smoking, drinking, and recreational drug usage are all noteworthy, and should be addressed. The mother's education level is not a necessary subject for the dietary counseling session.

33. D: Vitamin A levels, which are necessary for proper retinal development, are higher in colostrum than in human or cow's milk. Vitamin D, which is necessary for adequate calcium absorption, is lower in human and cow's milk than in colostrum. Supplementation with vitamins or sunlight exposure is needed to provide additional vitamin D. Human milk has lower amounts of vitamin K than cow's milk. Vitamin K levels, necessary for proper blood clotting, are lower in human milk than in cow's milk.

34. D: Breastfed infants need 200 IU of vitamin D per day and an iron supplement. All newborns should receive vitamin K orally or IM to prevent coagulation problems. All preterm infants need vitamin/mineral supplementation.

35. E: Age six months is a good time to introduce solid foods into the infant's diet. At this age, the infant has depleted the reserved iron stores, which need supplementation from age four months. The infant, at age six months, can produce IgA to discourage absorption of food

antigens that might cause allergies. The infant has the chewing and swallowing reflexes that allow them to eat food from a spoon.

36. E: Breast milk contains several bioactive components that defend the newborn infant against infection and boost the development of the immune system. Human milk and colostrum contain secretory IgA, immunologically specific cells, enzymes, carrier proteins, and hormones. Secretory immunoglobulin A (sIgA) and secretory immunoglobin M (sIgM) protect the gastrointestinal tract mucous membrane against the invasion of pathogens. There is no evidence of breast milk influencing the lymphocyte production of the newborn.

37. C: Human milk provides antibacterial protection by means of antibodies, the bifidus factor, lactoferrin, oligosaccharides, immunomodulators, and lactoperoxidases. The bifidus factor, a carbohydrate found in human milk and colostrum, sustains the growth of Lactobacillus bifidus. Lactobacillus bifidus is a beneficial strain of bacterium, which promotes antibody production and restores normal flora balance. Lactoferrin is a protein that binds with iron needed by pathogens such as Escherichia coli and Candida albicans and prevents them from proliferating. Lactoferrin also promotes the proliferation of T- and B-lymphocytes. Lactoperoxidase is an enzyme that, in combination with IgA, kills Streptococci.

38. C: The major causative agents of mastitis are Staphylococcus aureus, Escherichia coli, and Streptococcus. Antibiotic therapy is indicated, and occasionally incision and drainage of the breast become necessary. Emptying the breast is insufficient treatment. Leukocyte levels of >106, bacterial counts of >103, and high salt levels are typically found in the diagnostic test results.

39. D: Respiratory distress syndrome (RDS), hypoglycemia, and inborn malformations occur at a higher rate in the diabetic mother's newborn.

40. D: Nicotine suppresses the let-down reflex, and smoking has been shown to lower milk volumes. Nicotine and its primary metabolite, cotinine, can be found in the milk of smoking mothers. Stop-smoking aids such as nicotine patches and nicotine gum release nicotine into the breast milk.

41. C: Breastfeeding may resume after 24 hours of antibiotic therapy in the mother with staphylococcal mastitis.

42. E: Fever, rash, hypotension, desquamation (flaking or peeling of the skin), and multiple organ involvement occur with maternal toxic shock syndrome (TSS). Nausea and vomiting may occur because of organ involvement, but tarry stools are not a common sign of TSS.

43. E: The clinician should explain to the mother with HCV that although the chances of transferring the virus are low, if it does occur, there are no vaccines or immunoglobulin preparations currently available for treating the infection. HCV may cause a chronic infection of the liver in the newborn. The CDC sanctions breastfeeding by HCV-positive/HIV-negative mothers, but HCV-positive/HIV-positive mothers can transmit both viruses through the breast milk. Infants of mothers who have HCV should be tested for alanine aminotransferase (ALT) levels until age 15 months, and HCV-RNA and anti-HCV at between 18 and 24 months.

44. D: Post mature infants, who remain in utero beyond the period of vitality of the placenta, often lose weight, subcutaneous fat, and stores of glycogen. They are frequently predisposed to hypoglycemia and may need IV therapy and have low calcium levels. During the delivery of the post mature infant, intrauterine hypoxia, which results from insufficient placental reserves, can lead to low O2 levels in the infant and possible asphyxiation. The result of this hypoxia is decreased motility of the intestinal tract and low hormone levels, which may lead to difficulty in suckling.

45. A: Jaundice occurs in many newborns shortly after birth. The American Academy of Pediatrics guidelines for treatment of hyperbilirubinemia are:
- Day two of life, if the total serum bilirubin (TSB) level is ≥ 12 to 15 mg/dL, phototherapy is considered
- Day three of life, if the TSB level is ≥ 15 mg/dL, phototherapy is considered
- For older neonates with TSB levels of ≥ 17 to 20 mg/dL, phototherapy is considered
- If TSB levels continue to rise and phototherapy is ineffective, exchange transfusion is instituted

46. B: Hyperbilirubinemia with jaundice occurs at around 5 to 10 days after birth and usually continues for up to 30 days. TSB levels of > 20 mg/dL, a history of the mother having had another infant with jaundice, or the jaundice lasting over one week are all factors that indicate that breastfeeding should be discontinued until serum bilirubin levels are tested and the effects of breastfeeding are determined. If TSB levels are moving up toward 15 mg/dL, increased efforts to decrease the bilirubin are necessary. These include more frequent breastfeeding sessions and stimulation of stooling and breast milk production (via pumping).

47. D: The symptoms of necrotizing enterocolitis (NEC) include abdominal distention, vomiting, diarrhea, and blood in the stool. Hematuria is not a common symptom of NEC. There is some evidence that colostrum and breast milk may protect against NEC.

48. E: "Milk fever" is a condition heralded by a brief bout with fever, chills, dejection, engorgement, and depression due to hormonal (prolactin) changes.

49. D: The Breastfeeding Attrition Prediction Tool (BAPT), Maternal Breastfeeding Evaluation Scale (MBFES), Breastfeeding Self-Efficacy Scale (BSES), the LATCH Breastfeeding Assessment Tool, and the Infant Breastfeeding Assessment Tool are all commonly used breastfeeding assessment tools and questionnaires.

50. E: The main tenets of the IBCLC scope of practice include giving capable, evidence-based care, upholding professional standards, promoting and supporting breastfeeding, providing expert services for the mother and family, maintaining records and reports, protecting privacy and confidentiality (do not discuss one patient's case with another patient), and proceeding with reasonable diligence.

Secret Key #1 - Time is Your Greatest Enemy

Pace Yourself

Wear a watch. At the beginning of the test, check the time (or start a chronometer on your watch to count the minutes), and check the time after each passage or every few questions to make sure you are "on schedule."

If you are forced to speed up, do it efficiently. Usually one or more answer choices can be eliminated without too much difficulty. Above all, don't panic. Don't speed up and just begin guessing at random choices. By pacing yourself, and continually monitoring your progress against your watch, you will always know exactly how far ahead or behind you are with your available time. If you find that you are one minute behind on the test, don't skip one question without spending any time on it, just to catch back up. Take 15 fewer seconds on the next four questions, and after four questions you'll have caught back up. Once you catch back up, you can continue working each problem at your normal pace.

Furthermore, don't dwell on the problems that you were rushed on. If a problem was taking up too much time and you made a hurried guess, it must be difficult. The difficult questions are the ones you are most likely to miss anyway, so it isn't a big loss. It is better to end with more time than you need than to run out of time.

Lastly, sometimes it is beneficial to slow down if you are constantly getting ahead of time. You are always more likely to catch a careless mistake by working more slowly than quickly, and among very high-scoring test takers (those who are likely to have lots of time left over), careless errors affect the score more than mastery of material.

Secret Key #2 - Guessing is not Guesswork

You probably know that guessing is a good idea - unlike other standardized tests, there is no penalty for getting a wrong answer. Even if you have no idea about a question, you still have a 20-25% chance of getting it right.

Most test takers do not understand the impact that proper guessing can have on their score. Unless you score extremely high, guessing will significantly contribute to your final score.

Monkeys Take the Test

What most test takers don't realize is that to insure that 20-25% chance, you have to guess randomly. If you put 20 monkeys in a room to take this test, assuming they answered once per question and behaved themselves, on average they would get 20-25% of the questions correct. Put 20 test takers in the room, and the average will be much lower among guessed questions. Why?

1. The test writers intentionally writes deceptive answer choices that "look" right. A test taker has no idea about a question, so picks the "best looking" answer, which is often wrong. The monkey has no idea what looks good and what doesn't, so will consistently be lucky about 20-25% of the time.
2. Test takers will eliminate answer choices from the guessing pool based on a hunch or intuition. Simple but correct answers often get excluded, leaving a 0% chance of being correct. The monkey has no clue, and often gets lucky with the best choice.

This is why the process of elimination endorsed by most test courses is flawed and detrimental to your performance- test takers don't guess, they make an ignorant stab in the dark that is usually worse than random.

$5 Challenge

Let me introduce one of the most valuable ideas of this course- the $5 challenge:

You only mark your "best guess" if you are willing to bet $5 on it.
You only eliminate choices from guessing if you are willing to bet $5 on it.

Why $5? Five dollars is an amount of money that is small yet not insignificant, and can really add up fast (20 questions could cost you $100). Likewise, each answer choice on one question of the test will have a small impact on your overall score, but it can really add up to a lot of points in the end.

The process of elimination IS valuable. The following shows your chance of guessing it right:

If you eliminate wrong answer choices until only this many answer choices remain:	Chance of getting it correct:
1	100%
2	50%
3	33%

However, if you accidentally eliminate the right answer or go on a hunch for an incorrect answer, your chances drop dramatically: to 0%. By guessing among all the answer choices, you are GUARANTEED to have a shot at the right answer.

That's why the $5 test is so valuable- if you give up the advantage and safety of a pure guess, it had better be worth the risk.

What we still haven't covered is how to be sure that whatever guess you make is truly random. Here's the easiest way:

Always pick the first answer choice among those remaining.

Such a technique means that you have decided, **before you see a single test question**, exactly how you are going to guess- and since the order of choices tells you nothing about which one is correct, this guessing technique is perfectly random.

This section is not meant to scare you away from making educated guesses or eliminating choices- you just need to define when a choice is worth eliminating. The $5 test, along with a pre-defined random guessing strategy, is the best way to make sure you reap all of the benefits of guessing.

Secret Key #3 - Practice Smarter, Not Harder

Many test takers delay the test preparation process because they dread the awful amounts of practice time they think necessary to succeed on the test. We have refined an effective method that will take you only a fraction of the time.

There are a number of "obstacles" in your way to succeed. Among these are answering questions, finishing in time, and mastering test-taking strategies. All must be executed on the day of the test at peak performance, or your score will suffer. The test is a mental marathon that has a large impact on your future.

Just like a marathon runner, it is important to work your way up to the full challenge. So first you just worry about questions, and then time, and finally strategy:

Success Strategy

1. Find a good source for practice tests.
2. If you are willing to make a larger time investment, consider using more than one study guide- often the different approaches of multiple authors will help you "get" difficult concepts.
3. Take a practice test with no time constraints, with all study helps "open book." Take your time with questions and focus on applying strategies.
4. Take a practice test with time constraints, with all guides "open book."
5. Take a final practice test with no open material and time limits

If you have time to take more practice tests, just repeat step 5. By gradually exposing yourself to the full rigors of the test environment, you will condition your mind to the stress of test day and maximize your success.

Secret Key #4 - Prepare, Don't Procrastinate

Let me state an obvious fact: if you take the test three times, you will get three different scores. This is due to the way you feel on test day, the level of preparedness you have, and, despite the test writers' claims to the contrary, some tests WILL be easier for you than others.

Since your future depends so much on your score, you should maximize your chances of success. In order to maximize the likelihood of success, you've got to prepare in advance. This means taking practice tests and spending time learning the information and test taking strategies you will need to succeed.

Since you have to pay a registration fee each time you take the test, don't take it as a "practice" test. Feel free to take sample tests on your own, but when you go to take the official test, be prepared, be focused, and do your best the first time!

Secret Key #5 - Test Yourself

Everyone knows that time is money. There is no need to spend too much of your time or too little of your time preparing for the test. You should only spend as much of your precious time preparing as is necessary for you to pass it.

Once you have taken a practice test under real conditions of time constraints, then you will know if you are ready for the test or not.
If you have scored extremely high the first time that you take the practice test, then there is not much point in spending countless hours studying. You are already there.

Benchmark your abilities by retaking practice tests and seeing how much you have improved. Once you score high enough to guarantee success, then you are ready.
If you have scored well below where you need, then knuckle down and begin studying in earnest. Check your improvement regularly through the use of practice tests under real conditions. Above all, don't worry, panic, or give up. The key is perseverance!

Then, when you go to take the test, remain confident and remember how well you did on the practice tests. If you can score high enough on a practice test, then you can do the same on the real thing.

General Strategies

The most important thing you can do is to ignore your fears and jump into the test immediately- do not be overwhelmed by any strange-sounding terms. You have to jump into the test like jumping into a pool- all at once is the easiest way.

Make Predictions

As you read and understand the question, try to guess what the answer will be. Remember that several of the answer choices are wrong, and once you begin reading them, your mind will immediately become cluttered with answer choices designed to throw you off. Your mind is typically the most focused immediately after you have read the passage and question and digested its contents. If you can, try to predict what the correct answer will be. You may be surprised at what you can predict.

Quickly scan the choices and see if your prediction is in the listed answer choices. If it is, then you can be quite confident that you have the right answer. It still won't hurt to check the other answer choices, but most of the time, you've got it!

Answer the Question

It may seem obvious to only pick answer choices that answer the question, but the test writers can create some excellent answer choices that are wrong. Don't pick an answer just because it sounds right, or you believe it to be true. It MUST answer the question. Once you've made your selection, always go back and check it against the question and make sure that you didn't misread the question, and the answer choice does answer the question posed.

Benchmark

After you read the first answer choice, decide if you think it sounds correct or not. If it doesn't, move on to the next answer choice. If it does, tentatively check that answer choice. This doesn't mean that you've definitely selected it as your answer choice, it just means that it's the best you've seen thus far. Go ahead and read the next choice. If the next choice is worse than the one you've already selected, keep going to the next answer choice. If the next choice is better than the choice you've already selected, check the new answer choice as your best guess.

The first answer choice that you select becomes your standard. Every other answer choice must be benchmarked against that standard. That choice is correct until proven otherwise by another answer choice beating it out. Once you've decided that no other answer choice seems as good, do one final check to ensure that your answer choice answers the question posed.

Valid Information

Don't discount any of the information provided in the question. Every piece of information may be necessary to determine the correct answer. None of the information in the question is there to throw you off (while the answer choices will certainly have information to throw you off). If two seemingly unrelated topics are discussed, don't ignore either. You can be confident there is a relationship, or it wouldn't be included in the question, and you are probably going to have to determine what is that relationship for the answer.

Avoid "Fact Traps"

Don't get distracted by a choice that is factually true. Your search is for the answer that answers the question. Stay focused and don't fall for an answer that is true but incorrect. Always go back to the question and make sure you're choosing an answer that actually answers the question and is not just a true statement. An answer can be factually correct, but it MUST answer the question asked. Additionally, two answers can both be seemingly correct, so be sure to read all of the answer choices, and make sure that you get the one that BEST answers the question.

Milk the Question

Some of the questions may throw you completely off. They might deal with a subject you have not been exposed to, or one that you haven't reviewed in years. While your lack of knowledge about the subject will be a hindrance, the question itself can give you many clues that will help you find the correct answer. Read the question carefully, and look for clues. Watch particularly for adjectives and nouns describing difficult terms or words that you don't recognize. Regardless of if you understand a word or not, replacing it with the synonyms used for it in the question may help you to understand what the questions are asking.

Look carefully for these descriptive synonyms (nouns) and adjectives and use them to help you understand the difficult terms. Rather than wracking your mind about specific detail information concerning a difficult term in the question, use the more general description or synonym provided to make it easier for you.

The Trap of Familiarity

Don't just choose a word because you recognize it. On difficult questions, you may not recognize a number of words in the answer choices. The test writers don't put "make-believe" words on the test; so don't think that just because you only recognize all the words in one answer choice means that answer choice must be correct. If you don't recognize words in all but one answer choices, then focus on the one that you do recognize. Is it correct? Try your best to determine if it is correct. If it does, that is great, but if it doesn't, eliminate it. Each word and answer choice you eliminate increases your chances of getting the question correct, even if you then have to guess among the unfamiliar choices.

Eliminate Answers

Eliminate choices as soon as you realize they are wrong. But be careful! Make sure you consider all of the possible answer choices. Just because one appears right, doesn't mean that the next one won't be even better! The test writers will usually put more than one good answer choice for every question, so read all of them. Don't worry if you are stuck between two that seem right. By getting down to just two remaining possible choices, your odds are now 50/50. Rather than wasting too much time, play the odds. You are guessing, but guessing wisely, because you've been able to knock out some of the answer choices that you know are wrong. If you are eliminating choices and realize that the last answer choice you are left with is also obviously wrong, don't panic. Start over and consider each choice again. There may easily be something that you missed the first time and will realize on the second pass.

Tough Questions

If you are stumped on a problem or it appears too hard or too difficult, don't waste time. Move on! Remember though, if you can quickly check for obviously incorrect answer choices, your chances of guessing correctly are greatly improved. Before you completely give up, at least try to knock out a couple of possible answers. Eliminate what you can and then guess at the remaining answer choices before moving on.

Brainstorm

If you get stuck on a difficult question, spend a few seconds quickly brainstorming. Run through the complete list of possible answer choices. Look at each choice and ask yourself, "Could this answer the question satisfactorily?" Go through each answer choice and consider it independently of the other. By systematically going through all possibilities, you may find something that you would otherwise overlook. Remember that when you get stuck, it's important to try to keep moving.

Read Carefully

Understand the problem. Read the question and answer choices carefully. Don't miss the question because you misread the terms. You have plenty of time to read each question thoroughly and make sure you understand what is being asked. Yet a happy medium must be attained, so don't waste too much time. You must read carefully, but efficiently.

Face Value

When in doubt, use common sense. Always accept the situation in the problem at face value. Don't read too much into it. These problems will not require you to make huge leaps of logic. The test writers aren't trying to throw you off with a cheap trick. If you have to go beyond creativity and make a leap of logic in order to have an answer choice answer the question, then you should look at the other answer choices. Don't overcomplicate the problem by creating theoretical relationships or explanations that will warp time or space. These are normal problems rooted in reality. It's just that the applicable relationship or explanation may not be readily apparent and you have to figure things out. Use your common sense to interpret anything that isn't clear.

Prefixes

If you're having trouble with a word in the question or answer choices, try dissecting it. Take advantage of every clue that the word might include. Prefixes and suffixes can be a huge help. Usually they allow you to determine a basic meaning. Pre- means before, post- means after, pro - is positive, de- is negative. From these prefixes and suffixes, you can get an idea of the general meaning of the word and try to put it into context. Beware though of any traps. Just because con is the opposite of pro, doesn't necessarily mean congress is the opposite of progress!

Hedge Phrases

Watch out for critical "hedge" phrases, such as likely, may, can, will often, sometimes, etc, often, almost, mostly, usually, generally, rarely, sometimes. Question writers insert these hedge phrases, to cover every possibility. Often an answer choice will be wrong simply because it leaves no room for exception.

Switchback Words

Stay alert for "switchbacks". These are the words and phrases frequently used to alert you to shifts in thought. The most common switchback word is "but". Others include although, however, nevertheless, on the other hand, even though, while, in spite of, despite, regardless of.

New Information

Correct answer choices will rarely have completely new information included. Answer choices typically are straightforward reflections of the material asked about and will directly relate to the question. If a new piece of information is included in an answer choice that doesn't even seem to relate to the topic being asked about, then that answer choice is likely incorrect. All of the information needed to answer the question is usually provided for you, and so you should not have to make guesses that are unsupported or choose answer choices that require unknown information that cannot be reasoned on its own.

Time Management

On technical questions, don't get lost on the technical terms. Don't spend too much time on any one question. If you don't know what a term means, then since you don't have a dictionary, odds are you aren't going to get much further. You should immediately recognize terms as whether or not you know them. If you don't, work with the other clues that you have, the other answer choices and terms provided, but don't waste too much time trying to figure out a difficult term.

Contextual Clues

Look for contextual clues. An answer can be right but not correct. The contextual clues will help you find the answer that is most right and is correct. Understand the context in which a phrase is stated. This will help you make important distinctions.

Don't Panic

Panicking will not answer any questions for you. Therefore, it isn't helpful. When you first see the question, if your mind goes blank, take a deep breath. Force yourself to mechanically go through the steps of solving the problem and using the strategies you've learned.

Pace Yourself

Don't get clock fever. It's easy to be overwhelmed when you're looking at a page full of questions, your mind is full of random thoughts and feeling confused, and the clock is ticking down faster than you would like. Calm down and maintain the pace that you have set for yourself. As long as you are on track by monitoring your pace, you are guaranteed to have enough time for yourself. When you get to the last few minutes of the test, it may seem like you won't have enough time left, but if you only have as many questions as you should have left at that point, then you're right on track!

Answer Selection

The best way to pick an answer choice is to eliminate all of those that are wrong, until only one is left and confirm that is the correct answer. Sometimes though, an answer choice may immediately look right. Be careful! Take a second to make sure that the other choices are not equally obvious. Don't make a hasty mistake. There are only two times that you should stop before checking other answers. First is when you are positive that the answer choice you have selected is correct. Second is when time is almost out and you have to make a quick guess!

Check Your Work

Since you will probably not know every term listed and the answer to every question, it is important that you get credit for the ones that you do know. Don't miss any questions through careless mistakes. If at all possible, try to take a second to look back over your answer selection and make sure you've selected the correct answer choice and haven't made a costly careless mistake (such as marking an answer choice that you didn't mean to mark). This quick double check should more than pay for itself in caught mistakes for the time it costs.

Beware of Directly Quoted Answers

Sometimes an answer choice will repeat word for word a portion of the question or reference section. However, beware of such exact duplication – it may be a trap! More than likely, the correct choice will paraphrase or summarize a point, rather than being exactly the same wording.

Special Report: How to Overcome Test Anxiety

The very nature of tests caters to some level of anxiety, nervousness or tension, just as we feel for any important event that occurs in our lives. A little bit of anxiety or nervousness can be a good thing. It helps us with motivation, and makes achievement just that much sweeter. However, too much anxiety can be a problem; especially if it hinders our ability to function and perform.

"Test anxiety," is the term that refers to the emotional reactions that some test-takers experience when faced with a test or exam. Having a fear of testing and exams is based upon a rational fear, since the test-taker's performance can shape the course of an academic career. Nevertheless, experiencing excessive fear of examinations will only interfere with the test-takers ability to perform, and his/her chances to be successful.

There are a large variety of causes that can contribute to the development and sensation of test anxiety. These include, but are not limited to lack of performance and worrying about issues surrounding the test.

Lack of Preparation

Lack of preparation can be identified by the following behaviors or situations:

Not scheduling enough time to study, and therefore cramming the night before the test or exam
Managing time poorly, to create the sensation that there is not enough time to do everything
Failing to organize the text information in advance, so that the study material consists of the entire text and not simply the pertinent information
Poor overall studying habits

Worrying, on the other hand, can be related to both the test taker, or many other factors around him/her that will be affected by the results of the test. These include worrying about:

Previous performances on similar exams, or exams in general
How friends and other students are achieving
The negative consequences that will result from a poor grade or failure

There are three primary elements to test anxiety. Physical components, which involve the same typical bodily reactions as those to acute anxiety (to be discussed below). Emotional factors have to do with fear or panic. Mental or cognitive issues concerning attention spans and memory abilities.

Physical Signals

There are many different symptoms of test anxiety, and these are not limited to mental and emotional strain. Frequently there are a range of physical signals that will let a test taker know that he/she is suffering from test anxiety. These bodily changes can include the following:

Perspiring
Sweaty palms
Wet, trembling hands
Nausea
Dry mouth
A knot in the stomach
Headache
Faintness
Muscle tension
Aching shoulders, back and neck
Rapid heart beat
Feeling too hot/cold

To recognize the sensation of test anxiety, a test-taker should monitor him/herself for the following sensations:

The physical distress symptoms as listed above
Emotional sensitivity, expressing emotional feelings such as the need to cry or laugh too much, or a sensation of anger or helplessness
A decreased ability to think, causing the test-taker to blank out or have racing thoughts that are hard to organize or control.

Though most students will feel some level of anxiety when faced with a test or exam, the majority can cope with that anxiety and maintain it at a manageable level. However, those who cannot are faced with a very real and very serious condition, which can and should be controlled for the immeasurable benefit of this sufferer.

Naturally, these sensations lead to negative results for the testing experience. The most common effects of test anxiety have to do with nervousness and mental blocking.

Nervousness

Nervousness can appear in several different levels:

The test-taker's difficulty, or even inability to read and understand the questions on the test
The difficulty or inability to organize thoughts to a coherent form
The difficulty or inability to recall key words and concepts relating to the testing questions (especially essays)
The receipt of poor grades on a test, though the test material was well known by the test taker

Conversely, a person may also experience mental blocking, which involves:

Blanking out on test questions
Only remembering the correct answers to the questions when the test has already finished.

Fortunately for test anxiety sufferers, beating these feelings, to a large degree, has to do with proper preparation. When a test taker has a feeling of preparedness, then anxiety will be dramatically lessened.

The first step to resolving anxiety issues is to distinguish which of the two types of anxiety are being suffered. If the anxiety is a direct result of a lack of preparation, this should be considered a normal reaction, and the anxiety level (as opposed to the test results) shouldn't be anything to worry about. However, if, when adequately prepared, the test-taker still panics, blanks out, or seems to overreact, this is not a fully rational reaction. While this can be considered normal too, there are many ways to combat and overcome these effects.

Remember that anxiety cannot be entirely eliminated, however, there are ways to minimize it, to make the anxiety easier to manage. Preparation is one of the best ways to minimize test anxiety. Therefore the following techniques are wise in order to best fight off any anxiety that may want to build.

To begin with, try to avoid cramming before a test, whenever it is possible. By trying to memorize an entire term's worth of information in one day, you'll be shocking your system, and not giving yourself a very good chance to absorb the information. This is an easy path to anxiety, so for those who suffer from test anxiety, cramming should not even be considered an option.

Instead of cramming, work throughout the semester to combine all of the material which is presented throughout the semester, and work on it gradually as the course goes by, making sure to master the main concepts first, leaving minor details for a week or so before the test.

To study for the upcoming exam, be sure to pose questions that may be on the examination, to gauge the ability to answer them by integrating the ideas from your texts, notes and lectures, as well as any supplementary readings.

If it is truly impossible to cover all of the information that was covered in that particular term, concentrate on the most important portions, that can be covered very well. Learn these concepts as best as possible, so that when the test comes, a goal can be made to use these concepts as presentations of your knowledge.

In addition to study habits, changes in attitude are critical to beating a struggle with test anxiety. In fact, an improvement of the perspective over the entire test-taking experience can actually help a test taker to enjoy studying and therefore improve the overall experience. Be certain not to overemphasize the significance of the grade - know that the result of the test is neither a reflection of self worth, nor is it a measure of intelligence; one grade will not predict a person's future success.

To improve an overall testing outlook, the following steps should be tried:

Keeping in mind that the most reasonable expectation for taking a test is to expect to try to demonstrate as much of what you know as you possibly can.
Reminding ourselves that a test is only one test; this is not the only one, and there will be others.
The thought of thinking of oneself in an irrational, all-or-nothing term should be avoided at all costs.
A reward should be designated for after the test, so there's something to look forward to. Whether it be going to a movie, going out to eat, or simply visiting friends, schedule it in advance, and do it no matter what result is expected on the exam.

Test-takers should also keep in mind that the basics are some of the most important things, even beyond anti-anxiety techniques and studying. Never neglect the basic social, emotional and biological needs, in order to try to absorb information. In order to best achieve, these three factors must be held as just as important as the studying itself.

Study Steps

Remember the following important steps for studying:

Maintain healthy nutrition and exercise habits. Continue both your recreational activities and social pass times. These both contribute to your physical and emotional well being.
Be certain to get a good amount of sleep, especially the night before the test, because when you're overtired you are not able to perform to the best of your best ability.
Keep the studying pace to a moderate level by taking breaks when they are needed, and varying the work whenever possible, to keep the mind fresh instead of getting bored. When enough studying has been done that all the material that can be learned has been learned, and the test taker is prepared for the test, stop studying and do something relaxing such as listening to music, watching a movie, or taking a warm bubble bath.

There are also many other techniques to minimize the uneasiness or apprehension that is experienced along with test anxiety before, during, or even after the examination. In fact, there are a great deal of things that can be done to stop anxiety from interfering with lifestyle and performance. Again, remember that anxiety will not be eliminated entirely, and it shouldn't be. Otherwise that "up" feeling for exams would not exist, and most of us depend on that sensation to perform better than usual. However, this anxiety has to be at a level that is manageable.

Of course, as we have just discussed, being prepared for the exam is half the battle right away. Attending all classes, finding out what knowledge will be expected on the exam, and knowing the exam schedules are easy steps to lowering anxiety. Keeping up with work will remove the need to cram, and efficient study habits will eliminate wasted time. Studying should be done in an ideal location for concentration, so that it is simple to become interested in the material and give it complete attention. A method such as SQ3R (Survey, Question, Read, Recite, Review) is a wonderful key to follow to make sure that the study habits are as effective as possible, especially in the case of learning from a textbook. Flashcards are great techniques for memorization. Learning to take good notes will mean that notes will be full of useful information, so that less sifting will need to be done to seek out what is pertinent for studying. Reviewing notes after class and then again on occasion will keep the information fresh in the mind. From notes that have been taken summary sheets and outlines can be made for simpler reviewing.

A study group can also be a very motivational and helpful place to study, as there will be a sharing of ideas, all of the minds can work together, to make sure that everyone understands, and the studying will be made more interesting because it will be a social occasion.

Basically, though, as long as the test-taker remains organized and self confident, with efficient study habits, less time will need to be spent studying, and higher grades will be achieved.

To become self confident, there are many useful steps. The first of these is "self talk." It has been shown through extensive research, that self-talk for students who suffer from test anxiety, should be well monitored, in order to make sure that it contributes to self confidence as opposed to sinking the student. Frequently the self talk of test-anxious students is negative or self-defeating, thinking that everyone else is smarter and faster, that they always mess up, and that if they don't do well, they'll fail the entire course. It is important to decreasing anxiety that awareness is made of self talk. Try writing any negative self thoughts and then disputing them with a positive statement instead. Begin self-encouragement as though it was a friend speaking. Repeat positive statements to help reprogram the mind to believing in successes instead of failures.

Helpful Techniques

Other extremely helpful techniques include:

Self-visualization of doing well and reaching goals
While aiming for an "A" level of understanding, don't try to "overprotect" by setting your expectations lower. This will only convince the mind to stop studying in order to meet the lower expectations.
Don't make comparisons with the results or habits of other students. These are individual factors, and different things work for different people, causing different results.
Strive to become an expert in learning what works well, and what can be done in order to improve. Consider collecting this data in a journal.
Create rewards for after studying instead of doing things before studying that will only turn into avoidance behaviors.
Make a practice of relaxing - by using methods such as progressive relaxation, self-hypnosis, guided imagery, etc - in order to make relaxation an automatic sensation.
Work on creating a state of relaxed concentration so that concentrating will take on the focus of the mind, so that none will be wasted on worrying.
Take good care of the physical self by eating well and getting enough sleep.
Plan in time for exercise and stick to this plan.

Beyond these techniques, there are other methods to be used before, during and after the test that will help the test-taker perform well in addition to overcoming anxiety.

Before the exam comes the academic preparation. This involves establishing a study schedule and beginning at least one week before the actual date of the test. By doing this, the anxiety of not having enough time to study for the test will be automatically eliminated. Moreover, this will make the studying a much more effective experience, ensuring that the learning will be an easier process. This relieves much undue pressure on the test-taker.

Summary sheets, note cards, and flash cards with the main concepts and examples of these main concepts should be prepared in advance of the actual studying time. A topic should never be eliminated from this process. By omitting a topic because it isn't expected to be on the test is only setting up the test-taker for anxiety should it actually appear on the exam. Utilize the course syllabus for laying out the topics that should be studied. Carefully go over the notes that were made in class, paying special attention to any of the issues that the professor took special care to emphasize while lecturing in class. In the textbooks, use the chapter review, or if possible, the chapter tests, to begin your review.

It may even be possible to ask the instructor what information will be covered on the exam, or what the format of the exam will be (for example, multiple choice, essay, free form, true-false). Additionally, see if it is possible to find out how many questions will be on the test. If a review sheet or sample test has been offered by the professor, make good use of it, above anything else, for the preparation for the test. Another great resource for getting to know the examination is reviewing tests from previous semesters. Use these tests to review, and aim to achieve a 100% score on each of the possible topics. With a few exceptions, the goal that you set for yourself is the highest one that you will reach.

Take all of the questions that were assigned as homework, and rework them to any other possible course material. The more problems reworked, the more skill and confidence will form as a result. When forming the solution to a problem, write out each of the steps. Don't simply do head work. By doing as many steps on paper as possible, much clarification and therefore confidence will be formed. Do this with as many homework problems as possible, before checking the answers. By checking the answer after each problem, a reinforcement will exist, that will not be on the exam. Study situations should be as exam-like as possible, to prime the test-taker's system for the experience. By waiting to check the answers at the end, a psychological advantage will be formed, to decrease the stress factor.

Another fantastic reason for not cramming is the avoidance of confusion in concepts, especially when it comes to mathematics. 8-10 hours of study will become one hundred percent more effective if it is spread out over a week or at least several days, instead of doing it all in one sitting. Recognize that the human brain requires time in order to assimilate new material, so frequent breaks and a span of study time over several days will be much more beneficial.

Additionally, don't study right up until the point of the exam. Studying should stop a minimum of one hour before the exam begins. This allows the brain to rest and put things in their proper order. This will also provide the time to become as relaxed as possible when going into the examination room. The test-taker will also have time to eat well and eat sensibly. Know that the brain needs food as much as the rest of the body. With enough food and enough sleep, as well as a relaxed attitude, the body and the mind are primed for success.

Avoid any anxious classmates who are talking about the exam. These students only spread anxiety, and are not worth sharing the anxious sentimentalities.

Before the test also involves creating a positive attitude, so mental preparation should also be a point of concentration. There are many keys to creating a positive attitude. Should fears become rushing in, make a visualization of taking the exam, doing well, and seeing an A written on the paper. Write out a list of affirmations that will bring a feeling of confidence, such as "I am doing well in my English class," "I studied well and know my material," "I enjoy this class." Even if the affirmations aren't believed at first, it sends a positive message to the subconscious which will result in an alteration of the overall belief system, which is the system that creates reality.

If a sensation of panic begins, work with the fear and imagine the very worst! Work through the entire scenario of not passing the test, failing the entire course, and dropping out of school, followed by not getting a job, and pushing a shopping cart through the dark alley where you'll live. This will place things into perspective! Then, practice deep breathing and create a visualization of the opposite situation - achieving an "A" on the exam, passing the entire course, receiving the degree at a graduation ceremony.

On the day of the test, there are many things to be done to ensure the best results, as well as the most calm outlook. The following stages are suggested in order to maximize test-taking potential:

Begin the examination day with a moderate breakfast, and avoid any coffee or beverages with caffeine if the test taker is prone to jitters. Even people who are used to managing caffeine can feel jittery or light-headed when it is taken on a test day.
Attempt to do something that is relaxing before the examination begins. As last minute cramming clouds the mastering of overall concepts, it is better to use this time to create a calming outlook.
Be certain to arrive at the test location well in advance, in order to provide time to select a location that is away from doors, windows and other distractions, as well as giving enough time to relax before the test begins.
Keep away from anxiety generating classmates who will upset the sensation of stability and relaxation that is being attempted before the exam.
Should the waiting period before the exam begins cause anxiety, create a self-distraction by reading a light magazine or something else that is relaxing and simple.

During the exam itself, read the entire exam from beginning to end, and find out how much time should be allotted to each individual problem. Once writing the exam, should more time be taken for a problem, it should be abandoned, in order to begin another problem. If there is time at the end, the unfinished problem can always be returned to and completed.

Read the instructions very carefully - twice - so that unpleasant surprises won't follow during or after the exam has ended.

When writing the exam, pretend that the situation is actually simply the completion of homework within a library, or at home. This will assist in forming a relaxed atmosphere, and will allow the brain extra focus for the complex thinking function.

Begin the exam with all of the questions with which the most confidence is felt. This will build the confidence level regarding the entire exam and will begin a quality momentum. This will also create encouragement for trying the problems where uncertainty resides.

Going with the "gut instinct" is always the way to go when solving a problem. Second guessing should be avoided at all costs. Have confidence in the ability to do well.

For essay questions, create an outline in advance that will keep the mind organized and make certain that all of the points are remembered. For multiple choice, read every answer, even if the correct one has been spotted - a better one may exist.

Continue at a pace that is reasonable and not rushed, in order to be able to work carefully. Provide enough time to go over the answers at the end, to check for small errors that can be corrected.

Should a feeling of panic begin, breathe deeply, and think of the feeling of the body releasing sand through its pores. Visualize a calm, peaceful place, and include all of the sights, sounds and sensations of this image. Continue the deep breathing, and take a few minutes to continue this with closed eyes. When all is well again, return to the test.

If a "blanking" occurs for a certain question, skip it and move on to the next question. There will be time to return to the other question later. Get everything done that can be done, first, to guarantee all the grades that can be compiled, and to build all of the confidence possible. Then return to the weaker questions to build the marks from there.

Remember, one's own reality can be created, so as long as the belief is there, success will follow. And remember: anxiety can happen later, right now, there's an exam to be written!

After the examination is complete, whether there is a feeling for a good grade or a bad grade, don't dwell on the exam, and be certain to follow through on the reward that was promised...and enjoy it! Don't dwell on any mistakes that have been made, as there is nothing that can be done at this point anyway.

Additionally, don't begin to study for the next test right away. Do something relaxing for a while, and let the mind relax and prepare itself to begin absorbing information again.

From the results of the exam - both the grade and the entire experience, be certain to learn from what has gone on. Perfect studying habits and work some more on confidence in order to make the next examination experience even better than the last one.

Learn to avoid places where openings occurred for laziness, procrastination and day dreaming.

Use the time between this exam and the next one to better learn to relax, even learning to relax on cue, so that any anxiety can be controlled during the next exam. Learn how to relax the body. Slouch in your chair if that helps. Tighten and then relax all of the different muscle groups, one group at a time, beginning with the feet and then working all the way up to the neck and face. This will ultimately relax the muscles more than they were to begin with. Learn how to breathe deeply and comfortably, and focus on this breathing going in and out as a relaxing thought. With every exhale, repeat the word "relax."

As common as test anxiety is, it is very possible to overcome it. Make yourself one of the test-takers who overcome this frustrating hindrance.

Special Report: Retaking the Test: What Are Your Chances at Improving Your Score?

After going through the experience of taking a major test, many test takers feel that once is enough. The test usually comes during a period of transition in the test taker's life, and taking the test is only one of a series of important events. With so many distractions and conflicting recommendations, it may be difficult for a test taker to rationally determine whether or not he should retake the test after viewing his scores.

The importance of the test usually only adds to the burden of the retake decision. However, don't be swayed by emotion. There a few simple questions that you can ask yourself to guide you as you try to determine whether a retake would improve your score:

1. What went wrong? Why wasn't your score what you expected?

Can you point to a single factor or problem that you feel caused the low score? Were you sick on test day? Was there an emotional upheaval in your life that caused a distraction? Were you late for the test or not able to use the full time allotment? If you can point to any of these specific, individual problems, then a retake should definitely be considered.

2. Is there enough time to improve?

Many problems that may show up in your score report may take a lot of time for improvement. A deficiency in a particular math skill may require weeks or months of tutoring and studying to improve. If you have enough time to improve an identified weakness, then a retake should definitely be considered.

3. How will additional scores be used? Will a score average, highest score, or most recent score be used?

Different test scores may be handled completely differently. If you've taken the test multiple times, sometimes your highest score is used, sometimes your average score is computed and used, and sometimes your most recent score is used. Make sure you understand what method will be used to evaluate your scores, and use that to help you determine whether a retake should be considered.

4. Are my practice test scores significantly higher than my actual test score?

If you have taken a lot of practice tests and are consistently scoring at a much higher level than your actual test score, then you should consider a retake. However, if you've taken five practice tests and only one of your scores was higher than your actual test score, or if your practice test scores were only slightly higher than your actual test score, then it is unlikely that you will significantly increase your score.

5. Do I need perfect scores or will I be able to live with this score? Will this score still allow me to follow my dreams?

What kind of score is acceptable to you? Is your current score "good enough?" Do you have to have a certain score in order to pursue the future of your dreams? If you won't be happy with your current score, and there's no way that you could live with it, then you should consider a retake. However, don't get your hopes up. If you are looking for significant improvement, that may or may not be possible. But if you won't be happy otherwise, it is at least worth the effort.
Remember that there are other considerations. To achieve your dream, it is likely that your grades may also be taken into account. A great test score is usually not the only thing necessary to succeed. Make sure that you aren't overemphasizing the importance of a high test score.

Furthermore, a retake does not always result in a higher score. Some test takers will score lower on a retake, rather than higher. One study shows that one-fourth of test takers will achieve a significant improvement in test score, while one-sixth of test takers will actually show a decrease. While this shows that most test takers will improve, the majority will only improve their scores a little and a retake may not be worth the test taker's effort.

Finally, if a test is taken only once and is considered in the added context of good grades on the part of a test taker, the person reviewing the grades and scores may be tempted to assume that the test taker just had a bad day while taking the test, and may discount the low test score in favor of the high grades. But if the test is retaken and the scores are approximately the same, then the validity of the low scores are only confirmed. Therefore, a retake could actually hurt a test taker by definitely bracketing a test taker's score ability to a limited range.

Special Report: Additional Bonus Material

Due to our efforts to try to keep this book to a manageable length, we've created a link that will give you access to all of your additional bonus material.

Please visit http://www.mometrix.com/bonus948/iblce to access the information.